14,000 things to be happy about.

14,000 things to be happy about.

THE HAPPY BOOK
BY BARBARA ANN KIPFER

ILLUSTRATED BY PIERRE LE-TAN

WORKMAN PUBLISHING
NEW YORK

Library of Congress Cataloging-in-Publication Data is available.

ISBN 978-0-7611-8180-4

Illustrations by Pierre Le-Tan

Workman books are available at special discounts when purchased in bulk for premiums and sales promotions as well as for fund-raising or educational use. Special editions or book excerpts can also be created to specification. For details, contact the Special Sales Director at the address below, or send an email to specialmarkets@workman.com.

Workman Publishing Co., Inc.
225 Varick Street
New York, NY 10014-4381

workman.com
thingstobehappyabout.com

WORKMAN is a registered trademark of Workman Publishing Co., Inc.

Printed in the United States of America

First printing October 2014

10 9 8 7 6 5 4

TO KYLE

TO KEIR

THANK YOU

To Peter Workman: I knew you were the right one. That's why I pestered you for 10 years. You were right about there being 14,000 things, even though you encouraged me to continue my list-making habit. Big thanks to Sally Kovalchick, Susan Bolotin, and Mary Ellen O'Neill for their superb editing, guidance, support, and patience.

I also want to thank my programmer colleague and friend, Bob Amsler, for his invaluable assistance.

To my sons, Kyle Kipfer and Keir Magoulas, and my husband, Paul Magoulas: There is no greater happiness than you.

This book represents 50 years of recording all the little things that make me happy. Paying attention to life—to its beauty, oddity, wonder—is what happiness is all about. Beginning in sixth grade with a tiny spiral notebook, I kept collecting and moving to larger notebooks and finally to a computer. Although my database is well over 145,000 entries now, this book encapsulates what there is to be happy about and appreciative of in life. Words, and the images they create, are a great source of pleasure and inspiration. Flip through this book to cheer yourself up, remind yourself to be grateful, maybe even find something to do or something to cook for dinner.

As you read through these pages, give yourself time to conjure up your own images—to reminisce, wish, dream, awaken. I hope you will find, as I did, that happiness comes from appreciating the little things in life.

A stream-of-consciousness list
blueberry muffins
easeful days, dreamless nights
going roller-skating on a Saturday
      morning with corny organ music in
      the background
social and emotional intelligence
beet and goat cheese salad
sniglets, made-up new words
cookies with candied cherries on top
corn-husking and pumpkin-rolling
saltwater taffy
snow peaches
pseudonyms, like Mr. Big
keeping on nodding terms with the person
      you used to be

networking in business

memories of the good things you ate in
your childhood

moonlit dances on summer beaches

cinnamon apple waffles with real maple
syrup, well-done bacon, fresh fruit,
coffee, and fresh-squeezed juice

what your computer's desktop
background says about you

bringing beauty and meaning into
others' lives

getting a really good haircut

all the greens of spring

always carrying a notebook

unbuttoning peas on the porch

catching escaped veggies with a roll

finding a diamond in the rough

spatterware pails

the aromas of a tobacco store

selecting ripe melons

boneless duck with plum sauce and
fried rice

commuter drinking cups

filling a vase with red and blue anemones

Rudolph the Red-Nosed Reindeer (movie)

holding your shoulders high

books of answers

the taste of cake batter

a fresh idea in an artist's mind

the pure joy of the sun

recovering a fumble
your favorite airport
high-gloss white paint
waking up early and having breakfast
    together outside
butter mints
flexitarians
formal terraced gardens
popcorn popping all over the room
the smell of northern air
what makes human beings uniquely
    human
the butterfly effect
tender, loving touches
the art in everyday life
face creams that soothe
mists and intrigue
coleus spilling out of a window box
finishing the last freezing and canning
    for the winter supply
bifocal contact lenses
a newly refinished gym floor
touring model homes
horses breathing ostrich plumes of air
budō, the spiritual foundation for
    martial arts
buying summer sandals
taking a sabbatical year
a whiff of your favorite spice
part of you always being a child

overcoming acalculia (inability to do
  basic math)
diamondlike stars
the buzz of a bumblebee
ginkgo and willow trees
papaya with lemon cream
a tight-weave sisal bag for knitting
  supplies
writing down three things you appreciate
  each day
serendipity
aerial views
a place of secret magic where nature
  alone quietly renews itself
incurable enthusiasm
friendly aliens from outer space
shop talk
construction paper
old-fashioned sock monkey dolls
Viennese coffee, ground each morning,
  filtered into a thermos, and garnished
  with a cinnamon stick
Olympic trampolining
poems (*ghazals*) by Rumi
Santa's Village, Dundee, Illinois
bacteria, most of which are
  harmless and many of
  which are beneficial
Gothic novels
when all systems are "go"

body stockings
sturdy stew in white bowls
the reasoning "because it's there"
a stalled car catching
when the lights come up
the soothing winter wind in the hemlocks
remembering when leaves were raked,
    jumped into, or burned and not put
    in plastic bags or giant vacuums
English-style breakfasts and dinners in
    a riverside dining room
cable-knit sweaters
things you don't have to work at to enjoy
New York City
feeling the damp freshness of a Cape Cod
    morning cool on your face
checking your fortune-cookie message
    to see how it matches up with your
    partner's
French's mustard
pool parties
buttering toast generously and
    immediately so that the butter
    melts and sinks in
getting a job
"Do not remove this tag under penalty
    of law."
cheeks all aglow with the outdoors
Wyoming: Yellowstone, geysers, bears,
    broncos, ranches, Old Faithful

tremendous kettles of soup on a
    potbellied stove
an animal doing a tuck-and-roll
the sensuality of a scalp rub
hearing a glacier calve
prizes you have won
basketball, anytime, anywhere
Mod Podge
ginned cotton
the keys to the kingdom
snappy salutations
cheering influences
hearing, "You're the best."
satin-paper ribbon curled into crisp flower
    shapes
a portable whirlpool for the bath
carpet shampoo
organizing time
getting 100 percent on the spelling test
Christmas ball ornaments that open to
    reveal smaller balls
Kennebunkport and Kennebunk, Maine
the poetry of Pablo Neruda
personally witnessing a happy event in
    history
sailing on Lake Michigan
an ideal picnic spot
Palm Springs, California
Angora cats
sleeping sprawled out on the bed

quick postcards
"Those who have . . . get."
having a person to miss
deep-dish pies
an umbrella in a microburst
that your first instinct is almost always
    correct
catching fish
kids climbing the backstop
watering your garden
the trade winds
a leader's words that stir a nation
Ball Mason canning jars
a widow's walk
thoughts while ironing
onion buns
colonial wick lanterns
sweet effervescence
the large glacial deposits that form on
    the insides of car fenders during
    snowstorms
Introverts Anonymous
a sauce bowl and ladle
8,760 hours in a year
the little things in life that really make
    your day go right
plastic dry-cleaning bags
driving under an overpass during a storm
the old American custom of serving coffee
    on New Year's Day

where writers, artists, and tourists gather
playing among big trees and rocks
sightseers in all types of garb
pink grapefruit with tons of sugar
listening for the sound of a key in the lock
gratefulness
assembly lines
cherry pie à la mode
the United States of America
life choices
dress shoes
getting warm by a fire or in your partner's
 arms with something to eat or drink
 after you've been in the rain or snow
rare and expensive books
the gap in the dressing room curtain that
 can never be completely closed
the din of traffic
interesting wooden house siding
a "Eureka" moment
organic matter that gets caught in the
 rough world of rock surfaces
a successful first attempt
the rainbow and sand colors of pretty hair
counting married years in dog years
Monopoly's nine most-landed-on spaces:
 Illinois Ave., B&O RR, Free Parking,
 Tennessee Ave., New York Ave.,
 Reading RR, St. James Place,
 Water Works, Pennsylvania RR

a lively conversation between plants
not worrying about having what everyone
    else has
pelicans preening
key lanyards
cooks' kitchen gardens
peppermint whipped cream frosting
clothes that move and breathe
white tiger cubs
split-second thrills
suit coats
pantry shelves loaded with jars of fruit
silences in chess games
the rising or setting of a star at sunset
a tinkle gate bell affixed to a gatepost
hot peach conserve, a bottomless
    coffeepot, and eggs served in
    individual skillets
your first time in a foreign country
cinnamon and slate-blue satins
knowing a true genius
returning library books
an unexpected message from someone
    saying something lovely to you
observant men
putting extra raisins in Raisin Bran cereal
T's and jeans
carrying groceries in a backpack
tying colorful ribbons around things for
    the fun of it

gut-spilling softballs

Kansas wheat

the act of entering a room and
forgetting why

things that stand the test of time

preparing your Christmas card list before
Thanksgiving

turning off your email for short intervals

wild roses, blush-pink and spicily fragrant
in the cool of the evening

absorbing nature's blessings

a sense of pleasure and pride in the
achievements of one's children

filling a glass bowl with fresh apples and
tangerines

Jamaica, Bermuda, or clamdigger shorts

learning a new sport

"Let me bring lollipops and confetti
and silly things and place them at
your feet."

for purple dye: black cherry bark,
cocklebur plant, dandelion root,
grape

your favorite exhibits at the zoo

diamond earrings

"Away in a Manger" (carol)

Starbucks caramel macchiato

kids and games

draft horses

taking a refresher course

digital thermometers
auction bidding paddles
the structure of things
oil boom towns
cat hammocks
rising early
sponge baths
workworkworkworkwork
hearing your children praised by others
the one leaf that always clings to the end
    of the rake
melting-pot experiences
hostess gifts
a crisp white shirt and blue jeans
an inspiration board
watching an old Nora Ephron movie
sports shorts
clouds and mist rolling over a mountaintop
headache medicines
tidings of comfort and joy
riding in the basket of a bike
balsamic vinaigrette
downloading music
bakery croissants
plastic bags for wet swimsuits
a charismatic TV weatherperson
giving your hands cold-weather first aid
going back to your hometown: visiting the
    schools you attended, favorite and
    memorable places

rereading specific passages and chapters
    when seeking inspiration
guarantees that don't run out the day
    before something needs fixing
sliced London broil with sautéed onions
    and melted cheese on rye
Chinese barbecued ribs
a state of continual becoming
getting the last soda in the vending
    machine
mountains flaming with red, orange,
    and purple foliage
triumphing over adversity
music boxes
having the dog taste-test your food
the art of following through
a bedroom library
light snow in March
a shingled water tower
the riddles of space and time
lobster ravioli
late Sunday breakfast
brick floors
Tahitian tans
waking up an hour early and meditating
    outdoors
spotting a city slicker
using nippers to break up big chunks from
    a tall, cone-shaped loaf of sugar
homey touches

reliability

laundry soap

charred hot dogs

the segue to a new career

throw rugs

the onset of a peaceful feeling

clean, spacious, joyous settings

oven fries

planning a rites-of-spring party

"Life is a great big canvas; throw all the
    paint on it you can." (Danny Kaye)

when padded shoulders were in

frosted-glass walls

two ground beef patties, special sauce,
    lettuce, cheese, pickles, onion on a
    toasted sesame-seed bun

vine-covered trellises

plants on windowsills

lavender-scented evenings

using an art horse

Circle Line tours

discovering something desired is within
    your price range

an enchanted cottage

natural-history dioramas

sea salt and vinegar potato chips

skit night at camp

the great art of sauntering

getting snow caked on socks and
    in jeans cuffs

fresh, organically grown foods

two seats together at a crowded movie

songs of the meadowlark

winding country roads leading past rustic
farms with weathered barns and
stone fences

painting a mural

dandelions and buttercups

warm firesides

successfully doing a headstand

making a life, not just a living

steamer clams, dripping with drawn butter

the beach in the fall

BLTs and potato salad

Rural, Indiana

imparting an aura of passion, childlike
innocence, and serenity

Porsche 911s

alkaline batteries

an elegant stone terrace where guests
drop by for baked goods and coffee

a stand for your unabridged dictionary

learning to batik

a blue-and-white pitcher filled with
jasmine or daisies

plastic cups with built-in straws

regional offerings on the menu

the click of a closing purse

belief in two opposing ideas at the
same time

crepe de chine
library tables
the symmetry of roof tiles
a room just for creating art
reading *The New York Times* and
    USA Today every morning
writing in your diary in a secret code
peach cream-cheese pie
hot-coal walking
achieving flow, a psychological state
    where you are fully immersed and
    focused on an activity or a task
filling the pet food bowl
Rhodes Scholarships
reasonably lengthened life spans
not having the fear of missing out
a restaurant with goats grazing on the
    grass-covered roof
fluorescent-bright food stores
presidential autographs
registered Morgan colts
apricot strudel
church bazaars
taking in a classic tearjerker rather than
    the latest foreign film
knowledge, even in its tiniest increments,
    being one of the few pleasures that
    really endures
putting a pumpkin on the porch and a
    wreath of dried flowers on the door

bread and butter with pots of jam
    and honey
the Dalai Lama's smile
yestreen: yesterday evening
a skin-care regime
the NFL
a night without you or your partner snoring
anchoring just off a sandy crescent down
    the creek and casting for pan fish
waiting with bated breath
the inner city
mixed greens topped with chunks of
    chicken, tomatoes, and sprouts,
    served with honey-mustard dressing
introductory courses and textbooks
old stock certificates
a secluded houseboat on Arizona's
    Lake Powell
the law of attraction
boiling water for coffee
a smile, a sunny day, an ice-cold Coca-Cola,
    and a best friend to share them with
patting the cat
baked squash stuffed with rice and flavored
    with cinnamon, nutmeg, and allspice
having the windows washed
the times when you feel you're the only
    two people in the world
striped ribbons
leaves starting to turn

buying flowers for home on Fridays
an arabesque of vines braiding the door
the unique smell of new Play-Doh
an orderly kitchen
heavy glass humidors with solid-brass lids
marbleized paper as drawer liners
words like *forthwith*
morning coffee and juice brought to the
      guest rooms
a beautiful ferry ride
sweater dryers
sun-touched shoulders
cats in between ripples of blankets
Fez, Morocco
beer cheese soup
people who wrap presents instead of
      using gift bags
team studying
scarf skirts
night crawlers
bay swimming
French cuffs
an aircraft's four forces
baking-soda deodorant and detergent
attaché cases
scrapbooking stores
reading a favorite magazine
creamed onions baked with a cheese
      topping
a seaplane base

a boy's first facial hairs
the Cubs' Bleacher Bums
waxing floors
living with the knowledge that you've
    done your best
going barefoot around the house
starched linens
salt packets
padded bicycle seats
curling up with a book while your partner
    is out playing golf or watching sports
    on TV
something to be enthusiastic about
the magic curl of waves
anyone who can master the cartwheel
a before-breakfast walk
a doctor saying you or a loved one
    will be okay
mountains: a canvas for clouds
field glasses and bird book by the window
spine-tingling views
snow in October
hedge mazes
rockers: Presidential, Windsor, Snowshoe,
    Whitley Bent Back
loving your gray hairs
a garbage plate of baked beans, home-
    fried potatoes, onions, hot dogs, and
    barbecue sauce with bread and butter
    on the side

old-fashioned summers
lining closet shelves with scented paper
reserving your own quiet corner
dried vegetables, hung upside down
    in bunches
challenging yourself with a jigsaw puzzle
    or game app
finger-combing hair
Speedy Gonzales
Bliss, New York
crabmeat with sherried cheese sauce
sweet smells that change with
    passing hours
knit shirts
Woodstock, the bird in *Peanuts*
payday
baskets of sticky buns, cornbread,
    brioches, and seed-capped rolls
jewelry design
ultramarine blue
the incredibly elated feeling on a
    college campus after a major
    sports victory
a standing clipboard
local bon vivants
"May all your troubles be lexicological
    ones." (Christopher Hampton)
tomato chutney, mango chutney, etc.
tall people
old-fashioned lemon pie

winter bringing long, silent nights to
    dream on
writing a book
the token speed-up done by pedestrians
    waved on by a vehicle's driver
the call and response of two birds
July being National Ice Cream Month
listening to the auctioneer
philtrum, the indentation between nose
    and upper lip
Minute Rice
an order of frijoles
finding a drive-in movie and watching
    from behind the fence
a talkingstock
pulling the curtains, putting on some
    music, serving your favorite cocktails,
    and dreaming about what it must
    have been like to sail to
    Europe a long time ago
Adirondack yellow birch
the first star quietly coming out
ultrasoft sleep things
resting under cool trees
compliments to the chef
not being embarrassed easily
online courses and degrees
having a passion in life
"Layla" (song)
the exhilaration of pure winter air

walking a good brisk mile
a private elevator to a dining room
the order of colors in a Life Savers
    candy roll
singing to the radio when you drive
Blackletter or Gothic script
very colorful and cleverly lit oil paintings
    and watercolors
escaping from civilization
"Have a nice day" from a checkout person
fruit crates holding old record albums
walking tours
making lists, from major life goals to
    dinner menus
romantic declarations written in the sand
lady ferns, maidenhair, wood ferns, and
    cinnamon ferns
behind-the-scenes editors
noting the tiny details of drawings
bubble coral
showing sensitivity and concern
oysters on newspaper, family style
for a happy marriage: never speak loudly
    to one another, unless the house is
    on fire
wide-mouthed toasters
writing a final sentence
farm trucks chugging into the square with
    loads of fruits and vegetables
forming a "mind map" from a key concept

being knee-deep in foam and icy saltwater
tucking kids in for the night
sweatsuits favored by the elderly
making a birthday special
the steely twang-and-kazoo of a
    red-winged blackbird
horse-show ribbons on the wall
selling lemonade from a big earthenware
    crock set up on a card table on the
    sidewalk
sleepaway camp
archaeology buffs
green or blue eyes and frosted hair
children singing
plant-encrusted walls
the one song you can play on guitar
the splendor of fall
when all your senses are engaged
finding clarity
turning on the porch light to watch an
    evening snow sift down
building a model car
a prepaid gasoline or phone card
mahogany bowls from Haiti
the hemidemisemiquaver,
    demisemiquaver, and semiquaver
sea-torn, largely uninhabited coastline
friendliness
Oxford cloth curtains
an electric presence lingering in the air

pot roast/mashed potato meals
the calm before the storm
ham carved into fine-grained slices
antique headboards and tall chiffoniers
     with brass handles
buying a used textbook at a college
     bookstore
when your hair stays where you want it
the Appalachian Mountains
big changes
that vacation feeling
little bits of kitchen knowledge
a joke that is not disparaging
barbecue pizza, made with shredded
     barbecued pork in a sugar-and-spice
     tomato sauce
an orangutan bargaining for treats from
     the zookeeper
the Sistine Chapel's frescoes
the rugby tradition of repairing after a
     match to the local watering hole
rainy leaves stuck like emblems on
     the walk
the "upper crust"
silicon chips
"Hound Dog" by Elvis
blueberry cake after lobsters
Oriental bowls with a fish motif
three-way lightbulbs
doing well on the SATs

a swirl-pattern crystal bedside carafe with
    glass top
gored skirts
writing a letter to the editor
open lines of communication
the quiet spirit of holiday music
railroad date nails
luggage that stands out at the airport
Winnie-the-Pooh, Christopher Robin,
    Kanga, Baby Roo, Tigger, Eeyore,
    Piglet, Rabbit, and Owl
croissants with country jam and crumpets
    with honey
kiteboarding and kitesurfing
potpourris of dried flower petals, herbs,
    and aromatic spices
books on posture, body language
getting stuck in a beanbag chair
kids saying "Micky D's" and "BK"
attending a party on the terrace of
    a penthouse
a carpet of wild strawberries
sun worshippers
making love after a fight
living healthily a long, long time
sapodilla, tasting like peach, pear,
    cinnamon, and honey
pinion- and juniper-covered foothills
conversing in many languages and accents
how lucky you are

upper New York State
planning a purse sale
bracelet-length sleeves
powder mitts
Ivory soap
eating stuffing with raisins
pineapple-ham skewers
conjuring metaphors
a smoke-blackened brick fireplace
Greenland, formally Kalaallit Nunaat
Maslow's hierarchy of needs
squeezing one more brushful out of
    the toothpaste tube
countrified furniture
home: a quiet and personal space
soft snickerdoodles
the marvelous lighting effects created
    by sky, sun, clouds, and moon
blue topaz
Bermuda onions
being a lexicographer
pickle pimiento sandwiches with mayo
football terms
after supper, lying on a blanket and
    watching the fire die out
an edging of pansies in front of an inn
someone whose lines you always want
    to steal
rubber toy animals
a Chinese junk (ship)

whipped potatoes, coleslaw, and
     homemade pies
Bunsen burners
elevators
a salad-and-relish buffet
reading glasses
wild mushrooms, dried and arranged
     in a wooden bowl
getting an "I Voted!" sticker
always looking people in the eye
on your lunch hour: listening to music,
     visiting a planetarium, ice- or roller-
     skating, going to a museum, dancing,
     shooting darts, going to the Y,
     learning a foreign language, taking
     a bus ride, visiting a health spa,
     taking a tour, meditating
chicken broth
winding alleys
flumadiddle (utter nonsense)
long winter weekends
decorating a flowerpot
getting a swing twisted and then untwirling
On Demand movies
"Life is short. Eat dessert first."
     (Jacques Torres)
chuck, the hole in a pencil sharpener into
     which the pencil goes
the sticky sweet steam of a sugar house
     boiling off

bluffing at poker
windjammer vacations
riding through the desert in a dune buggy
squirting someone with a squirt gun
window sashes
familiar surroundings
jalapeño poppers
short ribs served in individual casseroles
     with sauce
waking up New Year's Day and knowing
     you didn't make a fool of yourself
the pinch marks on the ends of hot dogs
a street map of your town
finding the last item in your size at the store
Palladian windows
a baby smiling in its sleep
snow swirls
dishwashers
paint-by-number kits
carving pumpkins
cotton velveteen jeans
Autograph Day at the end of the
     school year
apple-glazed beef brisket
kick or punt, the indentation on the
     bottom of a wine bottle
giving a speech
Beethoven symphonies and sonatas
the purple of heather and yellow of gorse
     that inspire the patterns of Irish tweed

correcting the autocorrect

disasters you have survived

the first kiss of the summer

the comparatively early retirement age
of NFL players

a well-balanced life

Shaker crafts

the 64 poems in *A Child's Garden of
Verses* by Robert Louis Stevenson

vacationing off the grid

olive orchards that slope down to fields
punctuated with clumps of cypress
trees

bright yellow yolks

a "where did you get that?" item

seasonal cleaning of rugs

Swedish or Dutch butter cookies

your body being eight times the length
of your head

rare blue gumdrops

a litter of fluffy puppies

a rabbit named Buns

short-legged beach chairs

getting through the last chilly,
housebound nights of winter

tying hand-me-down sweaters around
your waist or neck

thick slices of radish, pepper, and
sweet butter on sliced French
baguette

all-butter pound cake, ice cream, and
    strawberries
the silence and solitude of isolated
    beaches
sticking with something you committed to
Wall Street
a yard of woolly thyme
good news for a change
eating peas with a fork
the bounty of nature
sandbox toys
the lawn settling into the sleep of frost
not hoarding
English muffins served with bacon and
    cheese
the hairdressing profession
putting together a swing set for children
    and seeing the look in their eyes
making sure you take your full vacation
    allotment
Wisconsin dairy products
eudemonics, the science of happiness
celebrating the imperfections of your
    relationship
the White Mountains
getting out the cashmeres and tweeds
the strains of the fiddle
a whale swimming with her calf
silent deserted shores
the roast carved, the corks drawn

café society
experiencing the thrill and sweat of
    a locker room
dimpling rains
previewing and ordering books online
simmering herbs and spices for good
    holiday smells
being all afizz
the freshest of ingredients, optimum
    in color, texture, and flavor
exploring a shipwreck
self-threading needles
people who brag that they never watch
    television but somehow know all
    the rules of the game shows
driver's education classes
living in a former gristmill
lessening the impact of a horror movie
    by filtering it through one's fingers
e.e. cummings, poet
being tall enough to reach
old medical or legal texts
lemon pound cake
diapers and baby food
Veronique Vienne's *The Art of Doing
    Nothing*
homemade *pain au chocolat*
cows with bells
a chemistry set to experiment with
cool limestone cellars

a white Christmas
Vietnamese cuisine
flodge, a small puddle
tiny satin pouch bags
having a picnic on the living room floor
chasing fireflies and talking in the yard
pipe racks
the spacious interior of a car
bicycling shoes
bacon frying in cast-iron skillets
jottings and musings preserved in one place
apricot refrigerator cake
Early American rockers
blanket, binoculars, hors d'oeuvres, and
   the top of a hill
the bottom line
traveling in the off-season
ice-cream cakes
the doughnut shop where everyone
   hangs out
browned turkey hash served with
   mustard sauce
sitting and watching a plant grow
remembering why you went into a room
an inherited book collection
looking your best
spending an afternoon skating or sledding
portable Scrabble games
an enameled coffeepot filled with
   dried flowers

cranberry juice cocktail
brick-paved residential streets with
    restored Victorian homes
being unfailingly faithful
one of those lucky days when there is
    a ton of stuff in the refrigerator
a celebration breakfast
yellow stacks of *National Geographic*
20 minutes all to yourself
cough lozenges
ducking into the ladies' room for ten
    minutes
a hypothesis
breaking out of an old routine
yin and yang
even-numbered ages sounding younger
freshly prepared soup
dill mustard
beating a video game
"The Farmer in the Dell" (song)
the plastic wand that launches
    soap bubbles
Old Sturbridge Village and the
    Publick House
city planning
tanning salons
choosing a new ensemble for
    a Barbie Doll
Vermont maple salad bowls
mischievousness

supermarkets
the roller derby
soft-lighting effects
being well-fed, well-exercised, well-read,
    well-rested, and well-paid
a vintage farmer's milk strainer
mysterious ploys
bluegrass fairs
wind-up animals
a quesadilla with jalapeños and a mojito
a paw in the fishbowl
switching to whole-grain bread
fuchsia, golden-warm marigolds, coral-
    to-magenta petunias, paper-white
    gardenias
Toll House cookie batter
drawing tablets
pea-planting day
crazy kids
warming milk for cocoa
bicycle shirts and shorts
laser printers
anagnorisis, the critical moment of
    recognition or discovery
conviviality
the duck motif
something sending your spirits soaring
high school rock bands
the smell of fresh-cut greens
beating the heat

a rainbow of ribbons

holiday soaps

the practice of eating the cream center
of an Oreo before eating the cookie
biscuit

variegated yarn and glimmer yarn

gleaming gold buttercups and wild
geraniums turning pink faces
toward the sunrise

50 percent off anything

jitney service

wheat fields

chocolate-covered cherries

watching a bridal party have pictures
taken

day headlights on cars

shop doorways

when friends drop in

when the February sky is gun-barrel gray

sleeping on the porch in summer

sugar wafers

local listings of lectures and panel
discussions

the sun coming up over a fog, a warmth of
silver light that seems to come from
everywhere

Ritz crackers

apple, peach, and fruit country

being an upperclassman

making love after tennis

what people are interested in, their
thoughts, the books they read and the
speeches they hear, their table talk,
gossip, controversies, historical sense
and scientific training, the values they
appreciate, the quality of life they
admire
white on the evergreens
planting seeds
driving up and down the main street
of town
mirrors inside closets
the potential of 45,000 words per pencil
two glasses of iced tea and a
bowl of cookies on a tray
the U.S. Air Force
Ionic columns
the visual language of comics
and cartoons
a pond or lake cupped in a
hollow among the green hills
the refrigerator egg holder
working as an umpire
a classic routine from vaudeville
wholesale boxes of Hershey bars,
Caramellos, and Tootsie Rolls
something that is one of a kind
allowing every guest to hang an ornament
on your Christmas tree
movable feasts

Porky Pig
getting asked out on a date early
mallards skimming low over the sea
political consciousness
kicking off your shoes and splashing your
	feet in a pool
listening to the lowing of cattle in a
	nearby field
the prow of a ship
freshly delivered French bread
a collection of hot sauces
a romantic walk through the neighborhood
	to look at Christmas decorations
beach rocks brought home in a backpack
	on your bicycle
Winnebago motorhomes
someone who wants to take you dancing
fruit peddlers
an off-the-cuff compliment
love, 15, 30, 40, game, set, match
enlarging a favorite photo
Betty Crocker cookbooks
the Earth's concentric layers
free concerts in the park
Lincoln wheat-cent coins
mixing yellow and red light bulbs
satyagraha, nonviolent resistance
rock crystal Christmas ornaments
old, old black-and-white snapshots
sautéed fresh mushrooms

licking a cake bowl
discovering a different route to work
hiding behind curtains
every seventh wave being a big one
dill or chive butter for corn
coleslaw and sliced apple or pear
    on a burger
"Do not disturb" signs
Dairy Queen posters and price lists
spring training
ringing the bell for doggy's dinner and
    doggy running to you
a desktop scarred from good use
children racing headlong into the water,
    joy splashing up around them
spam and ad blockers
staples in the stapler
fresh fruit pancakes
a bow-back Windsor chair
filling tartlet shells
ticket windows
unpretentiousness
buttercream frosting
a sky the shade of faded blue jeans
bobbing for apples
knowing it's never too late to learn
barrel-jumping
smiling your smile
popcorn at the movies
colored fireplace logs

lighthouses
baskets of shells on a low table
riding in a caboose
clam cakes and chowder
an analytic approach
fried mozzarella and marinara sauce
haunted houses
having a different kind of sandwich
    for lunch
clouds with silver linings
flat griddles
a wind on the way when there's a red sky
    at sunset
a romance between a French shop girl
    and a Yale dropout
secondhand stores
making a TV commercial
museum lectures
Wilson Sporting Goods
cream cheese with chives spread on rye
    cocktail bread
sautéed eggplant slices
Adam and Eve
submitting a sealed bid
itching after playing in the snow
a wish box
dessert picked off trees
nutmeg and Worcestershire sauce
    sprinkled on London broil or
    flank steak

jumping into bed with a good book
visiting a law school
Bermuda's pink beaches
the *Oxford English Dictionary* and its
supplements and the *Shorter Oxford
English Dictionary*
juicy barbecued delights
sidewalk hitching rings for horses
blueberries, pine cherries, woodbine,
raspberries, cranberries, honeysuckle,
wild roses, and beach plums
a perennial garden, thick with summer
bloom
anything you can get out of your system
or get closure on
people who have a will
changing a college major
log fires and feasts
slow snowfalls
maple-blueberry corn cake
a mockup of a website redesign
a psychic nudge that can widen your
perceptions
playing possum
Old Saybrook, Connecticut
getting fresh fish from someone who just
caught them
skating across a lake you swam in last
summer
using your powers for good

digging a hole in mashed potatoes to keep
    the gravy in
illegible handwriting, called griffonage
Sunday school
fajitas: a sizzling platter of charbroiled
    meat served with soft flour tortillas,
    cheese, tomato, lettuce, sour cream,
    and salsa
finding a pretty spot to sit and read the
    newspaper
love between two people
an antique pie cupboard
words like *akimbo, ennui,* and *salmagundi*
classic Spritz cookies
being taken to the zoo
the designated driver
rapturous organ music
gaming tables
scented oils
rural remoteness
happy songbirds
some really special and fitting words
    at Thanksgiving dinner
hot-water heating systems
winding a maypole
digging into baked apples
the weathered shingles of fishermen's
    shacks
freshly laundered jeans
old maps from a museum gift shop

the convenience of plastic or paper cups
open-air flower markets
"10-4" and other CB talk
seven brass candlesticks in graduated
    heights
secret civilizations
chipping in for a birdie
hard sauce over plum pudding, gingerbread,
    Indian pudding, or apple pie
wild violets growing profusely and making
    the prettiest of small bouquets
spoon bread
scoring super-high on a Scrabble turn
Swiss chocolate cake
a sense of humor in bed
a shore dinner
fueling a hot-air balloon
Tootsie Roll lollipops
an ice-cream truck with a tinkling bell
    and comet's tail of kids
cleaning soft-shell crabs
snow forts
wearing a smartwatch
little boys with froggies
scented soaps in dresser drawers
virga, rain that does not touch the ground
unsolvable Zen koans
an authentic Irish wool tweed tie
short-rooted spearmint and peppermint
    plants

banning all weapons and destroying all
    that exist
a kaleidoscope of colors
owning a lasagna server
love-knot rings
lying motionless in the warm sun
the 56 signers of the Declaration of
    Independence
squirrels hoarding nuts
the tradition of going to church on
    Christmas Eve
a matriarch
photojournalists and entertainment
    journalists with integrity
the individual vegetables or Tater Tots in
    a TV dinner tray that escape over the
    wall into the Salisbury steak zone
sequella, a secondary consequence
flipping coins into a fountain
knowing when to leave
the feeling that you're in a totally
    different world
classical music concerts
Difficult, Tennessee
poached white peaches
pizza samples
the first day of winter
things that taste, smell, feel, sound,
    and look wonderful: the stuff that
    romance is made of

old suitcases as coffee tables
the morning room, a quiet
    center of the home
challenging your own assumptions
coffee, light and sweet
accepting a compliment
charcoal-broiled fish
deep red dogwood and sourwood, yellow
    birch and beech, orange sassafras and
    bright red maples
chili sprinkled with strong chopped
    onions and triangles of cheese
home-garden varieties of squash, beans,
    and potatoes
Arthurian mythology
chic boutiques
rented tuxedos
Hefty plastic trash bags
your favorite ice-cream topping, indoor
    activity, Internet site, island
fishing with bamboo poles
the thirst-quenching deliciousness of real
    lemonade
herding reindeer and eating with the
    Lapps in northern Scandinavia
ketchup and mustard pump dispensers
Sharpie pens in every color
steep-walled, water-filled quarries
old wavy glass panes
G.I. Joe action figures

tranquility

chefs' outfits

paisley, plaid, cabbage-rose chintz
   wallpaper

carhops and OrderMatics

sending the sheets out to the laundry for
   wrinkle-free bliss

21st-century explorers

backpack-style handbags

the riverboat era

a mother calling to her child

the pleasure of discovery

the last pickle in the jar that resists being
   captured

walks along long piers

your team playing in the World Series

scones, delicious when served warm,
   split, buttered, and spread with jam

vata, pitta, kapha

barn houses

Frosted Flakes cereal

turkey trots

hanging lace curtains for an airy, open-
   window look

wooden ice-cream sticks

a shopping spree

a towel warmer in the bathroom

Brookstone gadgets

tropical fruits: cherimoya, Chinese
   grapefruit, kiwi, mango, and papaya

honey

satin vests

Victorian furniture and lamps with red bows

assisting a caterer

reading menus

rainy days, ideal for special projects
you've been procrastinating about

making concrete

putting shoes inside a shower cap before
putting them in luggage

crossword puzzle-ese

Saturday night dances

a clever paraphrase

singing songs around a campfire

serving sliced vegetables and fruits in
large wine goblets for dunking

door handles

the beat of a drum

a classic picnic of cheese and fruit

knowing one great idea can revolutionize
your life

tubing: bobbing in an old inner tube lazily
down a tranquil river

friendly Midwesterners

apples, trees, country sky, the snap of fall
in the air

being mistaken for a celebrity

the snowshoe hare turning white

astrology, numerology, tea leaves, crystal
balls, dice, tarot cards

sweet-potato soufflé with miniature
marshmallows and raisins
sour-cherry jam
wonderful-smelling dryer sheets
a big brother reading to a little brother
a gadfly
remembering when life moved at a more
leisurely pace
maple oatmeal muffins
keeping a child's heart happy
burning a Yule log only halfway, saving
the rest to light in the new year
enjoying what you reap from clearance
sales
feeling loved on Valentine's Day
round steak cooked on skewers
"That's the ticket!"
brand-new pencils
birthstones: garnet, amethyst, bloodstone
or aquamarine, diamond, emerald,
pearl or moonstone, ruby, sardonyx
or peridot, sapphire, opal or
tourmaline, topaz, turquoise
or zircon
a flea-market bin of antique photos
cold feet under blankets
a stimpmeter, used to measure the speed
of the greens on a golf course
Christmas music
adjustable hairbands

Dots candy
sparkling nonalcoholic grape juice
something as pretty as a picture
lobster tails baked individually in pastry
    with mushrooms and butter and
    served with wild rice and a vegetable
broadening someone's horizons
hand-tied fishing flies
treating yourself to a massage
learning the Latin equivalents for things
    you say all the time
mosquito zappers
small, sun-drenched houses overlooking
    a bay
Virginia jumbo peanuts
a giant cookie (cakie) for someone's
    birthday
seasoning with herbs instead of butter
    or oil
dish towels hung on cup hooks
piling tea sandwiches in a pyramid
comfortable old shirts as pajamas
the glint and glitter of frost crystals in the
    air, dancing like diamond dust in the
    sunlight
deep-set windowsills
a romantic scavenger hunt, steering your
    lover to a restaurant or back home for
    a private celebration
overcoming scaredness

fishing licenses
samba contests and confetti-showered
    parades
sliding glass doors
portable drafting tables
Google
fortune cookie: "To love and be loved is to
    feel the sun from both sides."
having good luck on a Friday the 13th
climbing on rainbows
happy endings
carving chicken or turkey
SpaghettiOs and franks
analyzing a blueprint
falling in love with an old friend
white grapes
the grayness of a sky about to snow
the art of cheesemaking
floating in tender clouds of silk
efficient couriers
"Your cake will brown slowly in the
    oven and rise like a perfect sun."
running a country store
the @ symbol
class reunions
a self-indulgent lunch all by yourself in
    a grand restaurant with a marvelous
    book as your companion
worn plush movie seats
a spa vacation

when your name is pronounced and
    spelled correctly
sprays of true-blue water
starting a collection
firm, moist, and crusty rye and
    pumpernickel bread
transoceanic airlines
talking sweetly
flickering gaslights
November's chrysanthemums
old photographs matted with small-print
    fabrics, a framed doily, and an old
    mirror
patchwork bench pads
gumball banks
smashing a piñata
the Blue Ridge Parkway, Virginia
looking through a very powerful telescope
the hobby of macramé
baskets from the harvest clustered on the
    kitchen steps
clip art
wrought-iron chandeliers
castles and fortresses
philanthropic billionaires
Montana: bitterroot, wind-sculpted buttes,
    snow, copper, sapphires, pasturelands
double boilers
dragonflies zipping
remembering which side the gas cap is on

the worn patch of ground under a swing
velour hooded sweatshirts
the hum of a motor
owning a watermelon baller
a window jungle of plants
spareribs spiced with herbs and honey
a cast-iron coffee mill
a class size of 20 or fewer
luggage that lasts a lifetime
the ability to start over
New York City publishing
correctly spelled and "clean" graffiti
a stuffed toy pig with piglets snapped on
advertising and advertisements
the windchill index and dew point
"You're never too old for Kool-Aid."
    (commercial)
pay dirt
enveloping yourself with calm; nourishing
     your senses and soul
the one who loves you
stone mansions
sweeping chimneys, taking up carpets,
     painting and whitewashing the
     kitchen, papering rooms; putting
     a new face on the house, in unison
     with nature
third basemen
indulging in an activity that isn't
     constructive or goal-oriented

when you wake up from a nap and
    realize time has barely passed
delicate ivory
when someone hurries up when you
    want him or her to
looking forward to your coffee break
    each day
history's years of insight
breakfast on the porch
long days at the beach
a sharp pencil
air terminals
apple wood burning in the hearth
taking a shower
the pseudo-meat, Spam
orthoscopic surgery
"The Night Before" by the Beatles
a sudden glimpse of a lit-up Christmas
    tree through a window
logical progressions
roving photographers
the croupier's rake for game chips
wrap coats
secret cabinets
kids who think bath is spelled y-e-c-c-h
pages softly turning
small, private weddings
a vinegary dressing with bits of bacon
European cheese
tablespoons

a string of ponies
coffee in a silver pot and
    a silver jug of hot milk
running your first mile
finding the doll of the
    child you used to be
luncheon orders
hand car washes that you wait in line for
being offered a football ticket
an herb-stuffed pillow
important trivia
free-form trees of glistening ice
ripe grass in need of comb and brush
beating people at Crazy Eights
calorie-intake control
energy taken out on a punching bag
recipes written at night
running after rainbows
butter curlers
liberation from grown-up routines
ferries to islands
kvelling
street food
counted cross-stitch
shorty skis
the wind whistling and moaning at
    the window and the stove with
    its steaming teapot sputtering a
    contented reply
cinnamon-brown birds

Monday Night Football
Denver, Colorado, and environs
striped canvas beach chairs
ignoring those who discourage you
free hot dogs
the noiseless flight of owls
Indiana Dunes State Park
razzmatazz
skinny ties
unsolicited spooning
a salmon-colored sunset
the yellowing pages of old books
blanket-checked fabric
rain showers
catfish and hush puppies
lighted swimming pools
shawl collars
reaching toward greater self-awareness,
    appreciation of beauty, and love of
    others
pullover tops
"The child that is born on the Sabbath day
    is bonny and blithe, and good and gay."
a green landscape
plain doughnuts
hearty soups straight from the stove
putting highlights in your hair
straightforward service
old, fancy two-piece pool sticks
irresistible softness

your favorite relative, rice dish, river,
    road sign, road trip game, rock
spray perfume
one true friend
snow-clad peaks
seashells in a glass bowl
the sound of the wind
school of spring: where little winds go
    to learn how to blow
Coleman stoves
roasting chestnuts in the fireplace
gourmet tools: oven rack push/puller,
    adjustable measuring spoon, bowl-
    fitting scraper, egg piercer, honey
    server, and strawberry huller
hour-long telephone calls
Hermagoras of Temnos, originator of
    using the five W's
buying a new mascara
putting perfume on your bike, in your
    hair, on your neck
country-manor breeding
silkworms, a domesticated insect
concerts on TV
snow patterns on windows
currant bushes hung with clusters of berries
a tall London oil lamp
Xerox copiers
Pisceans
soapbox derby racing

a county fair wheeling by in a Technicolor
    blur of sawdust and cotton candy
wave-splashed beaches
when you officially become a boyfriend
    or girlfriend
enormous bundles of Sunday newspapers
    on street corners
a recurring good dream
drivers who use their turn signals
checking the lotto numbers
chicken drumettes marinated with
    spicy sauce
doing something that will put a smile
    on your face
Polish sausage
spoiler alerts
arcipluvian: like a rainbow
the victory in good work
sexy high heels
wandering on brick-paved lanes lined
    with 18th-century houses
the vibrant colors of a Haitian painting
babies burping
helpfulness
being first-come first-served
a trapeze on a swingset
two-toned sports jackets
taste buds coming alive as you savor the
    smells of fresh-baked bread, fresh
    fish, and sizzling steaks

being able to fix your own toaster
"April Fool-ing is to end at noon, anyone
who tries it later is the fool."
when it is better that things did not work
out the way you wanted them to
spring collections of clothing
organizing images in an album
cowboy bars
prestige school activities: hall monitor,
honor committee, yearbook staff,
newspaper editor, athletic team
manager
a backless sundress
the blogosphere
one-day hikes
when the worst player scores
sculpture in papier-mâché
the seashell, symbol of good fortune
the books you plan to write
skier's suntan
Brie, Camembert, Havarti, and
Samso cheese
blue chambray work shirts
when you finally remember where you
recognize a person from
drive-in trays hooked onto windows
Clovis points
a job lot
the munching of a herd of sheep
frosty glasses

an open fire and the hearth on which
    it burns
pink lemonade
graph paper
apple pandowdy
Danish swirled pastries
a sociable personality
He shoots! He scores!
a reputation for the best food in town
P's and Q's, pints and quarts
going to sleep with a line through every
    item on the to-do list
an authentic lobster bake
manger scenes
when your temperature is at its 24-hour
    low: the time for your deepest, most
    restorative nap
icebox pinwheel cookies
wildflowers alongside a highway
a pushcart lunch
the discovery of a vocation
the quieter you become, the more
    you can hear
Dr. Seuss books
the three-day weekend
reviving tired furniture
a birdhouse shaking with activity
a January night that engraves itself on
    the senses
rich and ruddy complexions

nosegays of dried flowers

a retreat from the outside world

knowing when to work and when to play

keeping a list of favorite names

remarkable things emerging from the smallest, most ordinary circumstances

attic rooms

being between extrovert and introvert, an ambivert

team jackets

being able to sample the icing on a new cake without leaving a fingerprint

garnishes for soups: crème fraîche, bits of crisp bacon, julienne strips of ham, grated cheese, sliced fried sausage, buttered popcorn, salted whipped cream, sour cream, lemon slices or wedges, chopped fresh herbs (dill, parsley, or chives), or sliced or grated hard-boiled eggs

the camera phone

looking out a bus window

sci-fi

flying midweek

milk glasses

inflatable boats

staying healthy when everyone else has a cold

the seven virtues: charity, faith, fortitude, hope, justice, prudence, temperance muffler scarves

Conestoga wagons

answer pages in the back of textbooks

making special efforts to get to know
each other better

eggs over easy with toast

falling in love with a brass bed on a trip
to Vermont

skeet shooting

a wood fire

lush green gardens that roll gently down
to magnificent pink sandy beaches

telling people you've been afraid of
exactly what you think of them
and having the situation get better

raisin bread pudding with fresh
lemon sauce

eight ball

bake shops

a bleep

striped chintz pillows

Jägermeister's 56 herbs, fruits, roots,
and spices

odd-shaped mirrors in honey-colored
wood frames

old-time radio shows

dog dishes that say "Good Dog"

wrapping a taffeta ribbon around the
waist of a white tunic or tying pastel
ribbons around a straw hat

ropes of shells
yellow highlight pens that don't bleed
    through paper
evening purses
wreaths of pinecones hanging on
    heavy doors
the language of flowers
a 4.0 GPA
fun flashcards
Spanish olives
helpful hints books
street merchants
the quack of a duck
young marrieds
gaining energy by exerting energy
the feminine mystique
Canadian bacon and egg sandwiches
shared experiences and private jokes
a swoon
a richly hued paisley ottoman
laughing out loud
a bridge reopening
your own butter cookies
hanging a lamp over the center of the
    dining room table
winter piles drifting over the road
Marjolein Bastin, artist
visiting a farm to see all the newborn
    baby animals
rainbow sherbet

sewing groups
begonia pink
blowing bubble-gum bubbles
a surprise bonus
unique baby toys
energetic volunteers
dropping a preoccupation with oneself
organic peanut butter
no entrance fee
wild orchids
a steak over charcoal
thinking for yourself
steam rising from a cluster of casseroles
kids riding in shopping carts
an enjoyable or cute nickname
airing your blankets and quilts on a line
in the yard, beating your rugs, and
taking down heavy curtains
not peeking into a cannon
spiced tea
a solid-oak Chinese checkers game
leaving spaces in your day to do
something spontaneous
the St. Louis (or Los Angeles) Rams
the I-think-I-can whirring of VW Microbuses
hickory-grilled duck
All Fools' Day
grape-stomping contests
secretly planting tulip bulbs all over the
neighborhood

hamburgers with mustard, lettuce,
    tomato, pickle, onion, cheese, and
    hickory sauce
sewing-machine stitches
an in-room hotel hairdryer when you've
    forgotten yours
putting on overalls and getting dirty
fried egg in a "frame"
taking a sailboat to nearby islands
winning a spelling bee
the Berkshire Mountains
an enameled breakfront gas range
cheap thrills
"Kum Bay Yah" (Bible camp song)
rainbows apologizing for angry skies
going out on a Saturday night and coming
    home sober, having had a great time
resort wear
balancing on one foot
a portable aluminum camp grill
a flourish
fruit-filled waffles
a relationship that magically burgeons
    after simmering for years
double-handled soup bowls
stoneware and breakfast fixings
your best bet
joining hands at midnight on New Year's
    Eve and saying a special prayer for
    the coming year

any sign that takes on a new meaning
    when a magnetic letter falls off
a beach mat that doubles as a tote
R and R and R and B
buying a wonderful piece of furniture
    and enjoying it for years
crossword puzzle books
a gentle telephone ring
interrobang, a combination of the
    exclamation point and question mark
early adjournments
the red, gold, and blue-silver leaf of wild
    columbine
Scotch eggs
fish fries
an oasis
saving trinkets like Cracker Jack prizes
    and fair prizes
pulse points
harp, the metal hoop that supports a
    lampshade
the millions of Styrofoam wads that
    accompany mail-order items
firefighting apparatuses
painting bedrooms yellow
crows gathering together
a party in a pasture, barn, or gravel pit
food thrills
an attic's forgotten curios
bowls of vegetables being passed

Hellmann's mayonnaise or Miracle Whip?
passing your driving test
your own spaghetti
snow bringing a redeeming silence
walking into your dreams and coming out
a new person
raising llamas or alpacas
books: high information density per
pound, excellent value
sun-loving prairie plants
Tidewater saltbox homes
very romantic things or people
bonfire colors
yard sales
Labradors that think they're lapdogs,
Great Danes that eat off tables,
golden retrievers digging huge holes
in the rose garden, and basset hounds
sunbathing by the road
building a birdhouse
a definition's parts: definiendum and
definiens
a meaningful kiss
what it is like being you
homemade French silk pie
your favorite dairy food, dancer, day of
the week, deli meat, department
store, dinosaur, direction to travel,
dishwashing detergent, Disney
character, doll, doughnut

greasy-spoon restaurants
misty Taoist brush paintings
a colorful windjammer sailing fleet
crayon-striped sheets
the drilling of a woodpecker
the Kennedy Space Center
making your free throws
things that might come in handy
munching marshmallows
the symphony of the wind
the abating of a nuisance
accordion decorations and lamps
not biting when a growl will do
Frank Sinatra records
deep purple miniature eggplants, with
stems and leaves attached, piled high
on a round wicker platter and placed
on a violet tablecloth with deep
lavender napkins
tough feet
basking in the spring sunshine
note-taking on your favorite pad
planting tulips at Thanksgiving
seeing the biggest evergreen tree of your life
farm cats
percale sheets
fire poles
red-dogging the passer
a sustaining hot breakfast on a cold
winter morning

a romantic train trip
making an animated movie
cleaning up your own mess
evening caftans
special children's menus
sitting in the dorm, philosophizing
    about life
burying the hatchet with an old friend
    with whom you had a falling out
dark blue Indian cotton
sawing boards
your favorite one-liner, one-word answer,
    opera, outdoor activity, one of the
    Seven Dwarfs
the most absurd item you try to sell at a
    tag sale
the Highland fling
sunshine and weekends
prizewinning playwrights
making cozy provision against winter
E.T.: The Extra-Terrestrial (movie)
treasure-hunting with a favorite youngster
plum tomatoes
new-recipe night
dress shirts
cleaning the birdcage
joining a health club and getting results
strolling in Sunday best after the
    noontime meal
Polartec gloves

moonlighting because you want to
apples and Cheddar cheese cubes
large biceps
the lawn of an old English country house
coffee steaming gently from the spout of a
    tall blue enamel pot with a hinged lid
toys on sticks at amusement parks
film noir
designing a brochure
eating samples at a warehouse store
antique maps
the ever-present temptation to
    divert and amuse yourself
atmosphere drenched in history
the branching in the rays of a tail fin
pencil asparagus
chimney sweeps
portable talismans
smelling roasted sweet corn as you drive
warm-windowed houses and frosted-
    roofed barns
the Adler Planetarium
the historical Sanskrit language
crazy and silly and weird times
a cat chirping when it's happy
people who pay Visa bills with MasterCard
chicken wings, celery stalks, and blue
    cheese dressing
parfait stripes
the Atlantic Ocean

churns, copper kettles, oak kegs, wash
pots, buggies, woodstoves, cider
presses, coffee mills, kerosene
lamps—all sold at the general store
the promise of untold adventure
building a banana split
the pricelessness of integrity
tomatoes, red and sweet
hearing your spouse brag about you
your favorite salad bar item, Santa's
reindeer, *Saturday Night Live* skit,
seat in the car, slang word, sock color
the line you draw on a check to prevent
someone from writing "and a million
dollars"
handbags with room for everything
Spanish rice
the moon on the snow
not just seizing the day but making
the day
uncovering a lost garden
zipper teeth
rock-n-rolling roller coasters
baked fruit compote in the winter
a small act of grace
kids making their own Valentine cards
a Parisian tailgate picnic with baskets of
charcuterie
hiring window washers
something said tongue-in-cheek

a won't-leave-you-hungry meal
hand-rolled and -cut pasta
renting and borrowing for parties
the clatter of cross-country skis being
    stacked in the corner
having two magical days with no
    conversation, only contemplation
singing "and many more" at the end of the
    "Happy Birthday" song
heading south once in a while
chatting with the handyperson
early morning golf
illuminated manuscripts
sherry, cheese, biscuits, and a Bette
    Davis golden oldie on a rainy Sunday
    afternoon
getting chills when new dictionaries are
    published
tweed, Shetland wool, pearls
small dinners
hydroponic produce
The Katzenjammer Kids (comic strip)
Victorian knickknacks
going rogue
curve-of-the-Earth vistas
a fisherman's sweater
sitting in a rocker, listening to the silence
    and reflecting
no line for the restroom
tiny juice cans

an old-time corn popper with rotary agitator
the teeny petals of the mountain ash
geek chic
the ability of parents to guide their small
    children around by the tops of their
    heads
church hayrides
effective stress management
flower-decked floats
reservation books at restaurants
the *Rocky* movies
being crazy about someone
lamb souvlakia
party sounds behind a door you're about
    to open
pomp
old-fashioned stick candy in jars
daisies and black-eyed Susans
carrying things
Sunday naps
tapping trees to make syrup
pockets full of mittens
ties the width of lobster bibs
tools you can't live without
Passover and Rosh Hashanah
a fait accompli
surprising someone with a special event
at a hotel, unpacking a romantic picnic,
    sprawling out on the bed, and
    listening to the quiet

being tickled pink
"Tonight" and "Maria" (songs from
     West Side Story)
a balcony resting in the top branches of
     an oak tree
class rings
Jack Frost and his magic paint pot
abandoning all civility and slurping the
     grapefruit juice straight from the
     bowl it's served in
keeping your hopes up
doing everything with flair and a sense of
     fantasy
discovering a new singer, dancer, actress,
     writer, restaurant, recipe
throwing rice at newlyweds
guests at Buckingham Palace
a table with pots of fruit-bearing plants
     placed on it
red plush establishments
a city focused on the arts
bladed grass: a forest of small spears
soaking down a dog and standing back as
     it shakes dry
heat lamps in bathrooms
secondhand compliments
being adamant
Pilates workouts
Phillips screwdrivers
Kobe beef

majuscules and minuscules
animal gymnastics
the bottom of the Grand Canyon
sleek limos
looking for the best and enjoying it
rooftop planters
the soothing sound of sprinklers
    or waves
being given a new lease on life
a wrist corsage
making do
getting up on a 10-foot ladder for theater
    scenery work
the real importances: the fundamentals
    with which you have to live
sand, sea, and sunset
two chimneys holding a house like
    bookends
grocery store clerks you become
    acquainted with
the chug-chug of fishing boats
a cactus as a reminder of summer
walking to the baseball field after school
a pagoda's stories, each smaller than the
    one below
easy-out ice-cube trays
an art book on a stand
a bag of doughnut holes
sliding on the floor in your socks
taping your own ankle

clear nail polish

dart boards

I: the most common word in conversation

the teacher you remember

taking a bus to a small town with an
interesting name and staying a few
hours to explore

a use for the pocket on pajama tops

picnics in the car

tromping around with a candidate

microwave cooking

writing paper

early snows "healing" the landscape:
no tracks, no muddied slush

your favorite warm-weather vacation,
water sport, way to eat ice cream,
way to fall asleep, way to get
someone's attention, way to make
money, way to wake up, weekend
getaway, wine, world leader

the Great Lakes

popcorn balls in plastic wrap tied with
ribbon

endless space to fly a kite, play Frisbee,
run, walk, or just sit and think

window seats at a restaurant

a roadhouse

starting a relationship with a feeling
of wonder at the uniqueness of the
other person

waking up naturally (no alarm), pulling
    on a comfortable robe, brewing some
    coffee, picking up the paper, and
    getting right back under the covers
pink cottages
disc golf
radish-and-crabmeat salad
"Worrying is like rocking in a rocking
    chair: it gives you something to do
    but it doesn't get you anywhere."
    (from the movie *Van Wilder*)
designing a website
windsurfing in Bora Bora
horses with snow on their backs
the mantras of cat paws
any reunion that goes well
good magazines in the waiting room
pick-up sticks
word processors
breakfast-in-a-basket
sun-drenched climates
extra rest
Irish soda bread on St. Patrick's Day
doing all that you can to be safe online
bulk groceries
incomprehensible good luck
getting a check from the insurance
    company
rereading *Zen and the Art of Motorcycle
    Maintenance*

taking your shoes off for a long car ride
portable desks
the splintery crack of new books
people who act like ultimate experts on
     a topic after having read one article
     in the newspaper
get-acquainted parties
rippling layers of color
harbor lights
corny things
stubborn spider plants
reading lamps that cast the perfect
     amount of light on the page
cast-iron pans
two people listening to each other
classic shirts
seeing a new path in the woods
completing a project while still in your pjs
     and feeling productive all day
an antique two-seater school desk with
     cast-iron legs and an inkwell
60 Minutes (TV show)
the churning hum of the washing
     machine—a splashy mechanical
     giggle with a grinding note—
     tossing its wet mass one way,
     resting and simmering, then
     tossing it another way
a worm farm
dusk-time twittering of swallows

tomatoes and bacon on toast, covered
    with melted cheese
the pounding of a hammer
giving snakes the right of way
slumps, grunts, buckles, Bettys, and
    pandowdies
ozone
grated peels of fruit
brightly striped sweaters
buying postage online and printing it out
putting all your senses to work
lending a hand
aluminum pie weights
the log-and-chink walls of an old cabin
the delicate hieroglyphics of raccoons and
    deer down by the creek
the business of the day falling into
    manageable perspective
tree farms
packing a frosted cake for a trip
pot stickers
Ohio: glass, pottery, steel, tires, mound
    builders, fertile fields
reversible rain slickers
pulling pantyhose out of the drawer and
    finding them run-, snag-, and hole-free
the discovery of stunning early Maya
    paintings
poetry that doesn't rhyme
time-tested friends

a conversation that starts with a book
roast pork
violet: eggplants, beets, blackberries,
    mulberries, plums, purple grapes
playing in a closet as a child
bunches of asparagus, tied with ribbons,
    in a basket
cubed potatoes fried in bacon fat, salt,
    and pepper
butterflies migrating
a big bag of Hershey's Kisses
water's capacity to take any shape
a storm tapering off
steel drums and street dancing
lush thickness
redwood forests and Spanish moss
finding the perfect hairstyle
desk accessories in country fabrics
Pyrex cookware
wishing for a new car
harp seals
the places jeeps can go
taking piano lessons and never practicing
tiny pumpkins
a high-placed government source
brown eggs, cauliflower, and white onions
    in a pale straw basket with a few
    bronze daisies
hand-cut lead crystal decanters
omelet pans

spreading light

a wood-paneled saloon

finding a hidden bay, a secret backwater,
an old harbor, or a deserted beach in
complete isolation

making new bookstore friends

thinking before you speak

calm tempos

socks folded in matching pairs

white birch logs in the fireplace in summer

a moot point

woodcuts of your own design

a wintergreen toothpick

enchantment

chicken and lobster served in a special
sherry sauce

shepherd's pie

a cat circling a spot three or four times
before settling on it

ziplining over the Amazon

computational linguistics

tenpins, duckpins, candlepins, fivepins,
skittles, and ninepins

taking advantage of Indian summer

bicycling out to look at the Scotch
heather, wood lilies, and wild roses
on the moors

a feeling of oneness

cheese in 40-pound wheels

meeting a quota with pride

the six sides of a snowflake
shumai and its dipping sauce
light-giving flecks of diamonds
a butcher-paper dispenser
Mexican jumping beans
the clangor of a fire truck
guaranteed free delivery
seeing *The Nutcracker Suite*
meteorologists and chiropractors
velvet cushions
pocket caddies for reading chairs
10- or 20-pound bags of apples
Mother's Day presents
the name "Kyle Brian"
Vermont Cheddar cheese
loving forever
framed calico appliqué pictures
doughnut-hole machines
your childhood clubhouse
the Sundance Film Festival
the wind picking up, blowing the trees
    around wildly, then rain starting to
    pour, pounding the surface of a lake
    and creating rivers in the dirt
the salt of the earth
seeing the awesome and eerie ruins of
    Pompeii
ecotravelers and ecojourneys
soft, puffy, foot-long breadsticks with
    Italian tomato sauce

learning all the words to the songs you
 usually hum or whistle
being glad you have each other
a patisserie window that stops you in your
 tracks
supporting actors and actresses
being lifted or moved out of harm's way
the perfect box or container when you
 need it
a spa day
the peace sign and the happy face
Boeing 727s and 747s
the one you dress up for
pork and apples coddled in a nostalgic
 ginger-raisin sauce and creamy corn
 pudding on the side
legendary lovers
food ads and labels from decades past
library carrels
handmade afghans
having a favorite book
 bound in leather
striking poses
cashmere V-necks
cracked corn for
 the chickens
bubble gum and hard candy pieces in bags
 of a 100 or more
the deep sigh of a baby before he or she
 drifts off to sleep

learning something new in each paragraph
of a book
outdoor craft exhibits
the crunch of a breaking nut
well-insulated oven mitts
peeling fruit
simple dinners made up of soups, salads,
and vegetable dishes
Silly Putty
whitening toothpaste
luxuriant meadows with wildflowers
an elegant military ball
vertical barren rocks
getting something done by giving it to a
busy person
the International Space Station
showing off collections
stage set design
the empty stretches of bun on either end
of a hot dog
doing your job like no one else could do it
root beer candy
Velcro catch
cast-off time when sailing
a kitchen pegboard storage system
the Brannock device
not trying to do everything at once
watch fobs
going for it lock, stock, and barrel
soup or chili in a bread bowl

Martini & Rossi Asti Spumante
piggy banks
the pong of a tennis ball
colorful stationery in the pigeonholes of
your desk
a dog's face when you say "walk" or
"treat"
a clean litter box
an old-time rocking horse
the porch welcome light
calm soccer moms and dads
finding the most luscious piece of fruit
you can and savoring it
flimflam, another word for nonsense
getting in the right line at the store
taking Friday off
having a moral compass
the device at intersections marked "push
to cross"
airtight stoneware jars with attached
wooden spoons
a romantic garden, an English perennial
garden, a traditional herb garden
finally getting your hair cut so it's out of
your eyes
your book of the moment
clamshells
the Parker House hotel in Boston
waking up refreshed in the morning
hot zabaglione

not eating when you're not hungry
family values
a warm, crackling fire
waterfront buildings
softening brown sugar
an antique railway switching signal
funny business
pleasure being life's major concern
wedding buffet suppers
succulent baked chicken or country ham
    accompanied by fresh-baked rolls
receiving intelligent answers
finger cakes
cordial remarks for passersby
the medieval city of Siena, which gave
    "burnt sienna" to the artist's palette
iced tea with mint sprigs in wineglasses
taking time off
flipping to the right page of a book on the
    first try
watering cans
a true synonym, which is rare
hammered copper
lines from favorite movies or poems
sighs and whisperings
a view of sailboats skimming the horizon
soaking up some extra memories
well-buttered crumpets
happy holidays
all-purpose flour

pan gravy

theatergoing

open-minded uncertainty

rice-basket planters

touching-the-sky, dreamy, ice-creamy
    times

knit bedspreads

V-formations of migrating geese

the eerie appearance and ascension of the
    bubble in a water cooler

making at least a thousand dreams come
    true

the polonaises of Chopin

earth-toned, rustic linens giving warmth
    to rooms in fall or winter

excelling in your chosen occupation and
    avocation

the wind brushing past you

mastering the backstroke or butterfly
    stroke

open-toed strapped wedge sandals

a huge set of Faber-Castell colored pencils

short shorts

browsing new-car lots

a unique glory

making friends with the police

a bed left guiltlessly, spontaneously
    unmade

saying yes . . . yes . . . yes

the concept of one size fits all

furniture woods
meat platters
spring dinner parties
picnicking by the pond
overcoming writer's block
cloud nine
working out a problem
people who offer you their seat
a forest sanctuary
Linde Stars: waltzing, six-rayed star rings
crepes stuffed with mushrooms and
 Gruyère cheese in Mornay sauce
this thing called love
Easter dinners
a refuge from the city with fine, flat
 beaches
food that mittened hands can grasp
handling the first few minutes when
 meeting someone new
binding books by hand
the sea offering an omnipresent rumble
stream-fishing for trout
contentment in listening to music and
 staring at a fire
curating an exhibition at a gallery
the world of words
animals of intelligence: porpoise, fox, pig,
 chimpanzee, orangutan, elephant,
 gorilla, dog, beaver, horse, sea lion,
 bear, and cat

a Bad Day Survival Kit
old-fashioned glass snow domes
giving your least favorite food another
    chance
flopping around in a wading pool
when you had seat belts installed in the car
winning an eBay auction
pig noses
Woods Hole Marine Biological Laboratory
weathered docks on tall stilts
picking a sanctuary in your home: a favorite
    chair with good books nearby, a spot to
    come to and relax all by yourself
coming out of the water to dry and toast
writing about whatever you think of
    (things you wish, say, dream);
    observing people and writing down
    what you think they think
four-slice toasters
gentle, warm afternoons created for
    tennis parties and games of croquet
the phrase "cut the mustard"
French fry frying baskets
the many shades of gray
wanderlust
printing out photographs of your last
    vacation from your digital camera
fans of the Chicago Cubs
accolades
mobile concepts

a gentle ringtone

the first scratchy, camphor-smelling wool
  sweater of the season

the Energizer bunny

cobalt-blue bottles

Missouri: Huck and Tom, rocky glens,
  Pony Express, watermelons

beating the odds for a change

tool kits

taking a snowmobile tour

planning a hot summer midnight supper
  on the beach or near a lake

the drone of a passing plane

steel bands

wearing an Indiana Jones–style fedora

long-buried feelings and memories

the patina acquired by leather jackets and
  gloves, loafers, and jeans

the habit of checking for change in every
  coin return you pass

touch football games

kayaks for rent

a grandfather clause

dreaming nice dreams

soft music

Warren Dunes State Park, Michigan

refreshing your eyeballs

ham sandwich sauce: sweet-and-sour red
  tomato gravy, redolent of cloves

baby showers

taking advantage of every nook in your
    house
peach, pear, raisin, and rum cheesecakes
a recipe for banana toast
"All that we are is the result of what we
    have thought." (the Buddha)
when small miracles occur
senior proms
wooden buttons
leaving something unsaid
red geraniums
sitting on a bench to watch the billowing
    sails of the yachts negotiating the
    sparkling blue waters of a harbor
rejoicing in time alone to catch up
a life-goals list
watching the same TV shows as someone
    even when you're not together
Spike, Snoopy's brother
steeples rising like stalagmites
a bobbing float
hair ribbons
grating cheese
uneven parallel bars
bed bolsters
hollow-stemmed pilsner glasses
Trix and Fruity Pebbles cereals
quiet meals
creating exotic life stories for people who
    walk by

corn blades drifting in the breeze
red sweatpants
cruising a coastline
the color, scent, and deliciousness of
    strawberries
checking the battery fluid
correcting a mistake
seedless grapes in sour cream and brown
    sugar
planting a tree
wearing white cotton
making love
miniature jellybeans
the season to be jolly: the end of football
    until the beginning of baseball
a turret-shaped study
a vanity license plate and a college decal
    on the back window
executing a perfect Eskimo roll while
    kayaking
car-wash fundraisers
playing a kazoo backward
winter scarves in a variety of colors
garage sale "antiques"
people who understand there's a lot to you
wood-burning fireplaces
Bach concertos
a cosmopolitan atmosphere
Flutophones (recorders) in third-grade
    music class

oval picture frames

a blanket rack

Tinkertoys, Play-Doh, Etch A Sketch, Fisher-Price corn popper, Lego blocks, Monopoly, Scrabble, and an Erector set

a twosome sitting close together

a single orchid fed by ice cubes

being nice to someone who bugs you

tying a friendship bracelet

benches in between rows of lockers

broiling meat or toasting bread on the top rack of a woodstove

outrageous banana splits

writing positive inspirational thoughts in a quotations book

a baby-powder back rub

playing pool

when your teacher uses your work as a good example

Cheddar cheese pancakes

chopping blocks

a personalized leather-bound diary

the very first present of Christmas morning

putting a button on the corner of your beach towel so you can pull it on as a cover-up

babies in backpacks

a communal meal

nothing making more sense in the
    summer than forgetting to be sensible
pop tents
learning things from books of questions
    and answers
giant popovers
colorful flower and produce markets
The National Enquirer
Philadelphia cheesesteak
the dizzy smell of fresh-cut hay
crossing the bridge when you come to it
benefiting from a change in your point
    of view
baby's breath flowers
everyone needing a little love
saying something that no one else would
    dare to say
remembering when the highway patrol
    didn't hide with radar at the side of
    the road
your oldest Christmas decorations
a drive-up mailbox
happy feelings emanating from the
    kitchen
onion soup topped with croutons and
    melted cheese
jogging on a carpet of leaves as the sun-
    dappled trail winds through a thick,
    hardwood forest
earning Brownie points

towel racks
sharpening your vision
a handsome park
free kittens
a tea cozy
antique buttons
wine tastings
stove filaments turning radiant red
swankiness
long sojourns
happiness coming in three ways:
     anticipation, realization, memory
when the sky is clear and clean, the air
     crisp, the wind free of dust
your ring size being the same as your hat
     size
the first snow falling silently through
     miles and miles of spruce
interludes
tying shoelaces
rinsing pantyhose in almond soap
a beautiful calfskin leather agenda
poetry in everything
walkabouts
ceramic glaze
secret recipes
American Express cards
working on a project
flames for boiling and baking, coals for
     broiling and frying

golden lion tamarins
platform shoes
Ice Capades
taking a course
campfires and campsites
dips, chips, and football
feeding a cow
beautiful children
a thermos lunch
dark and cushy carpeting
baked pineapple
your favorite takeout food, tea flavor,
temperature, tennis partner, texture,
Thanksgiving food, thing to debate,
thing to do after work, thing to do
on a weekend, thing to doodle, thing
to put on after a shower, thing to do
while waiting
finding seats in a crowded movie theater
slabs of homemade fudge
coffee and doughnuts, their outsides
crisp and sugary, their insides light
and spicy
when you finally remember the word or
name you had on the tip of your tongue
discipline in exercise, food choices, and
self-care
expositions and fairs
wearing water wings in the bathtub
one rose in a tiny bouquet of wildflowers

investigating underwater
singing in the shower
thick woolen blankets
a Brobdingnagian cut of prime rib
sun-dried tomatoes, steamed shrimp,
     pasta, and pink sauce
not missing a thing
the colors of oatmeal
candied apples, pickled beets, buttered
     potatoes, string beans, and a half-
     dozen hot biscuits served with a
     pitcher of honey
Bartlett's Familiar Quotations (book)
the turbulent surface of the sun
excavating a kitchen midden
falling leaves
evaporating handwashing liquid
variations on the periodic table theme
saved money
snow on the weekend
chameleons seeing in two different
     directions at the same time
pints of Guinness
shin pads
boathouses
a black sweater with khaki pants
class acts
the last day of school
the spot on the shopping mall map
     marked "You are here"

eternity rings
ham salad on Canadian white bread
velvet Queen Anne chairs
handing out invitations
playing blackjack or 21
using your time to cultivate gardens
giving a soft answer to a not-so-soft
    question
lucidity in times of confusion
Arabian horses
a teacher who learns from students
shells in a shadow box
the klunk-klunk of a windshield wiper
a luxurious hotel bathroom with Jacuzzi,
    twin showerheads, and bathrobes as
    soft and enveloping as comforters
a boost when you most need it
effective business meetings
English library ladder chairs
escargot, cheese fondue, beef
    bourguignon, veggies with dips,
    and chocolate fondue with fresh
    fruit and angel food cake
the dynamics of a black hole
heated swimming pools
shy goldfish
Caribbean bartenders
being especially partial to book-lined
    rooms
the poetics of lists

herbed cottage cheese with a toasted
      bagel
write-in-the-dark pens
a robin's 3,000 feathers
your summer jobs
gingerbread houses outlined in white
      spun sugar, peppermints, candy corn,
      jellybeans, and gumdrops
a farmhouse-turned-restaurant
"Wash me" instructions found on the
      backs of dirty trucks
the odor of explosive powder from
      firecrackers
time to think things over
a warm mix of vegetables
being too busy to notice trivialities
a basket filled with strawberries, cherries,
      and green grapes
an odd couple
"I'd rather play tennis than cook." (slogan)
a vending machine accepting your dollar
painting your nails fire-engine red
strip steak with a tender, charred crust,
      plump and pink, packed with juices
square-legged redwood plant stands
the sea of phones recording the
      elementary school performance
the icy green sky at the horizon,
      pink/blue above, and near the
      zenith—a half-moon

bargain prices
online reference
barbecuing meat and vegetables
   summer-style on a cold winter night
   in a fireplace
having someone to come home to
highly polished parquet floors
plump white berries on mistletoe
church bells pealing, lights going on, and
   a festival beginning
the smell of a baby's skin
clear, cool alpine breezes blowing on
   steep, snowy mountains
sports video games
a radio pouring out a little Haydn quartet
the yacht club
luminarias to light a walkway
clothesline rope
a blue ribbon won at a playground
   pet show
college dormitories
tabletop mirrors
fans when you need them
orange segments
laughing at cringe-worthy
   things Mom said
white enamel coffee mugs
meats garnished with parsley and small
   red tomatoes
designated bike lanes

hand-blended larch and lemon potpourri
	in an embroidered pillow
the snowscape of a whitewashed house
fabric rosebuds
summer research projects
handkerchief linen
a cast-iron farm bell
pasta makers
a bowl of matches from watering holes
	around the world
what your desk thinks about at night
binoculars and notebooks
cleaning up accumulated dribbles of
	office or house work
Aunt Jemima syrup
a taste bud's life span of seven to
	ten days
a G-force simulator
a river trip on a sternwheeler
bachelor's buttons
an early hunting owl winging close
cream satin furniture
ripe plums
curtain calls
looking at all the colors you can see on
	a cloudy day
brushing your teeth in the shower
an espresso "slushy"
hot wax for your snowboard
the whirr of hummingbird wings

recording trivia and fact bites that
   interest you
painting the ceiling sky blue
Twelfth Night punch: apple cider, pineapple
   and orange juices, cinnamon, cloves,
   nutmeg, honey, ginger
the student union
the local Zen center
Fleet Street, London
coconut palm, mango, banana trees
many candles on a table
izzard: the archaic name of the letter *Z*
great human happiness
vegetables boiled in a huge kettle over an
   open hardwood fire
biking around campus
a broom-swept beach house
water pumps
stone rubbings
putting the cover over the birdcage at night
using a telephoto lens
attic junk
tearing out a piece of perforated paper
   perfectly
chickadees weighing as much as a first-
   class letter
paintings sold straight from the easel
buckwheat mix
lying down on the grass and following a
   cloud across the horizon

reversible place mats
pound cake and milk
butter-steamed carrots
learning a new word
lobster salad on split wiener buns
enthusiastic book reviews
the school nurse
babies wearing jeans
getting lots of sleep
a profession other than your own that you
	would like to attempt
little faces punctuated with the round o's
	of wide eyes and open mouths
eau de cologne
secret doors
Vermont scrambled eggs served with local
	Cheddar cheese
a steaming pot over a crackling fire
snuggling up with gentle creatures
the peal of an organ
happy times
exotic coral seashell and barnacle clusters
when dinners came with a sprig of parsley
	and a cracker basket
short socks
a whiff of peppermint
showing a dog
blueberry pancakes made with stone-
	ground whole-wheat flour, granulated
	sugar, whole milk, and blueberries

drawing tables
shaggy Dartmoor ponies
giving back
Hank Aaron, baseball player
laughing to keep from crying
artists who come to paint a scene and stay
on to open studios and galleries
manicured hands
two or three cabbages opened like flowers
in a basket
a fortiori, a posteriori, a priori
a porcupine, half asleep up in a big pine
when that first cup of coffee kicks in
blue lightbulbs
steaks sprinkled with fresh herbs
saying "Sure"
plants and shells as centerpieces
Herefords standing knee-deep in lush
grass
The Brothers Bloom (movie)
a baby's quilt
handed-down Christmas ornaments
the loon's distinctive white necklace in
contrast to its black plumage
peppermint-stick ice cream with whipped
cream topping and fudge in a small
pitcher on the side
rope railings
large scrapbooks
personalized golf balls

paying attention to the sounds of each
of the different instruments in a
symphony
popping salted peanuts
waterproofing your shoes
stopping to think about how you wish
it could be and realizing how good
you've got it
the Academy Awards
seeing someone you love do something
outstanding
Sandwich glass knobs
wild cherries
learning word roots
the individual squares of a waffle
squirrels building nests low in the trees
"moo" cows
Tibetan handbells
rain on a thirsty Iowa field
100 acres of mountaintop with a saltbox
house in New Hampshire
gardenias and candlelight
frozen yogurt
a third opinion
your favorite jam flavor, James Bond
movie, jazz singer, Jell-O flavor,
jellybean color, juice
the history of a four-poster bed
drafts scurrying like mice about the house
windows with tinted glass

throwing a pot

truck headlights that invade your motel room at three in the morning

the difference between achievement and aptitude tests

Gray's Anatomy, 1858 edition

finding lyrics on the Internet

regatta stripes

cream cheese and watercress triangles

when you think you're a kid again

feeling the warmth of the sun while sitting in a car on a cold day

long light glowing on a crusted meadow

the impossible encounters that live in the imagination and somehow become reality

golf clubs

a copper-and-brass coal scuttle used for kindling or small logs or as a sewing caddy

straw-blown paintings

natural and organic foods markets

Mexican seven-layer dip

a sushi chef's eye for aesthetic detail

washing your hair in rainwater

having orange juice and champagne while wearing silk pajamas

bookworming

happily impoverished students

word-of-mouth: a dish we find irresistible

hobby shelves
the writings and etchings on school desks
"Pronto!"
home projects
Peru's Machu Picchu
a thick mattress pad, soft feather pillows,
fresh flowered sheets, a cotton
comforter, and lace bed skirt
when a hamburger can't take any more
torture and hurls itself through the
grill into the coals
loving thy neighbor
one day's accomplishments that make up
for the previous week's interruptions
a bright, cheerful breakfast room
doing something against all odds
believing in yourself when no one else will
going up on the roof and examining your
neighborhood
peas amandine
curtains whispering
joie de vivre
someone loving the smell of your skin
New Hampshire primaries
wire baskets
swim meets
Salieri and Mozart, composers
keeping an eye out for UFOs
potato knishes
"Keep on truckin'" (saying)

a synchronized chorus line or swim team

driving by the house in which you grew up

seasonless corduroy, cotton gabardine,
    velour, denim

"As a man thinketh in his heart, so is he."
    (Proverbs)

cellophane noodles

miniature golf

van Gogh

pyramids of fruits and vegetables
    arranged in stalls

credit cards

handsome Georgian and Greek Revival
    mansions

November clouds, high, gray, and passing

bocce balls

American cheese

condominiums

buying soap bubbles and blowing them at
    an unsuspecting person

the iPad

a team of chefs

drop-leaf tables

blunt-tipped scissors, paper, and crayons
    for a child

a train huffing and puffing out of the
    station

trying something you haven't before, like
    an artichoke or a pomegranate

election signs on front lawns

an evenly lighted room to reduce
  eyestrain
choosing a watermelon
being motivated by self-knowledge
rubber-tipped doorstops
the art of reading faces
your life, turned into a hit sitcom
Fleetwood Mac
low wood beams
hanging clean, dry towels in your bathroom
a reawakened curiosity about nature
good advice
omelet-making
pioneer ways
tiny carafes
40-hanger coatracks
doing something spontaneous on a
  snow day
narrow-ruled paper
lush trees
Snoopy standing on a beach ball
wafer cookies
"Oooh doggies, the hoggies
  are out!"
just-right-length necklaces
a smooth transition
Irish linen place mats
an enameled pierced-steel pie keeper
turning cartwheels, doing headstands and
  somersaults

old-fashioned kitchens
sharing being something you like to do
bread boutiques
getting rid of unused electronics
cereal parties
railroad ties
raisins drying in the sun
odd utensils like an hors d'oeuvre fork,
    mini ladle for dressings and sauces,
    nut and berry spoon, olive and pickle
    fork
gadding about
the National Register of Historic Places
choosing a chandelier
stirring up warm, friendly feelings on a
    cold morning
using paper bags, not plastic—or better
    yet, a tote
a bubble of quiet air
sitting in the kitchen with your hands
    wrapped around a hot cup of coffee
    and musing on your life
braised short ribs and apples in cider
    sauce
dainty French daisies
the retort "Don't make me laugh!"
being spoiled
a baited hook
driving on an empty road
catching the breeze in a hammock

fresh flowers, crisp vegetables, hot
     popovers, hearty portions, lots of
     bath towels
back doors: the ones best friends enter by
the headlight on a vacuum cleaner
folding auditorium chairs
swell smells
hearing a brooklet gurgling and making
     bewitching sounds under the snow as
     it goes to join the waters of the pond
water sports
vegetable sauces: butter, hollandaise,
     Mornay, polonaise, sour cream,
     mustard, vinaigrette, white, or cream
multicolored file folders
a window shade that allows itself to be
     pulled down, hesitates for a second,
     then snaps up
painted turtles
the boxed area on a U.S. map where the
     49th and 50th states are located
woodchucks so fat they waddle
idea exchanges
for blue dye: blueberries, elderberries,
     indigo plant, larkspur flowers
white sand
trapezoids, pentagons, hexagons,
     octagons
waxy rubbings from scratched-off lottery
     tickets

hot dog stands
patching and sealing a driveway
white asters, pale as dry champagne
listening more than talking
remembering when bubble gum cost
a penny, comic books a dime,
hamburgers a quarter, and water
was free
discovering a niche market
cabana boys
daffodils looking like a carpet of yellow
transmission fluid
an antique lace hankie
the contagious act of yawning
bright sun causing you to feel sleepy
a C average not being the worst thing
epistemology, theory of knowledge
working toward goals
Old English lettering
meeting friends
strolling troubadours
errant clouds chasing each other across
the blue sky
making toast the old-fashioned way: on
the end of a toasting fork over flames
roaring in the fireplace
listening to Tchaikovsky's *Swan Lake*
wooden curtain rods and brackets
a rocking chair in front of a window
overlooking a lake

drinking wine from jelly jars
meat that is buttery textured, tender like
    pot roast
pails of first-run sap
tiny ice-cream stores
the smell of peat moss
gel pens
ten most beautiful words: *chimes,*
    dawn, golden, hush, lullaby,
    luminous, melody, mist,
    murmuring, tranquil
invigorating walks through forests or
    fields
whiter-than-white angel food cake
100-watt eyes
bowling leagues
backyard screen houses
watching people eat corn chips
vintage Coach handbags
Geiger counters
herbs and plants used for yellow dye:
    alder leaves, apple bark, aster
    flowers, bayberry leaves, chamomile
    flowers, horse chestnut husks, catnip,
    peach bark
mustard and dill sauce
the first few snowy mornings of any
    winter, wonderful and crisply
    beautiful
English rose potpourri in a jar

rolls and honey
uproarious laughter that must be
    forcibly squelched due to its
    inappropriateness in a situation
studying seed catalogs
believing that crying is good for you
mountain daisies at 11,000 feet in the
    Rockies
wood carvings
sunshine filtering through hanging plants
cats not holding grudges
noontime visits
passing a car safely
summer storms
leis placed on visitors to Hawaii
papaya, avocado, cucumber, snow peas,
    chives, and green onion salad with
    mint vinegar
mirror neurons in the brain
saying yes more than saying no
elegant tea services
not being required to do jury duty for
    another five years
starchy white fabric
tearing home from work to finish a book
Brunswick stew
firing a salute
free books
senior year
breakfast toast

a land bridge like the Bering Strait or
    English Channel
Saks Fifth Avenue
a Hawaii license plate on the mainland
grilling a steak
painter's pants
cider presses
falling asleep to music
volunteering as a cuddler for premature
    infants
wine cellars
What to Expect When You're Expecting
    (book)
yellow raincoats with hoods
helping others
carte blanche
the return of plain white Keds, the yo-yo,
    clove chewing gum
a distinguished professor
Amish quilts in a double wedding ring
    pattern
voicing your opinion where no one can
    hear you
a gigantic breakfast at Denny's
playing in autumn leaves
esoterica, singular things, done by a
    small group
sitting up straight
lunch and milk money
special people

viewing every problem as an opportunity
for learning new things
dinner menus
an aging flowerpot
meeting in the park for a touch football
game
sunup and sundown colors
a baby's yawn
chasing evil spirits away
carrying field guides in the trunk
kindred souls
something as fresh as candy mints
reading outside on a blanket wearing a big
sweater in the autumn sun
French fries cooked in duck fat and
served with aioli
Sierra Club hikes
still having a turntable for vinyl records
being gung ho
woodland paths
the Bhagavad Gita
coffee-colored kitchen appliances
wandering the fairgrounds, watching
demonstrations of making soap,
Christmas ornaments, and apple
fritters
someone dependable and solid with
dimples
the whole kit and caboodle
renting a convertible on vacation

comparative adjectives like snugglier-
    snuggliest, more-most
stapling the top of paper-bag lunches
breathtaking skating over transparent ice
serving flaming bananas for dessert
shearling fleece
multihued vineyards
avocado trees
burning calories while resting
Oktoberfest celebrations
ski pants
hunks of cheese in plastic wrappers
providing a breakfast of croissants or
    warm rolls, good jam, sweet butter,
    hand-squeezed orange juice, an egg
    dish; ham, sausage, or country bacon;
    and good coffee
miles of ribboned highway tied with
    cloverleaf bows
night sports
black lights
eating everyone's discarded pickles
a sympathetic ear
making colored, layered sand or salt jars
pressed-tin ceilings, arched doorways,
    and a winding stairway
cast-iron floor registers
Diners, Drive-Ins and Dives (TV show)
improving eating patterns
wearing earmuffs

checklists

putting up the storm sashes, checking the woodpile, and making sure the oil tank is full

footed bowls

crispy wontons with roasted red pepper and walnut dip

your inner hum

modern art

earthquake-proofing

clearing your head

a tapestry-and-hardwood Victorian rocker

runnels of condensation on the panes

"Rain before 7, done by 11."

a Scottish thistle-design shortbread mold

bootie slippers

taking off to a place you've never seen before

guardian angels

the *Mayflower*

water mains

white-painted bamboo

searchlights at fairs and festivals

orange soda

Shaker cabinets and cupboards

hot-water-method iced tea

the chapel choir loft, an excellent nook for making out

chicken Kiev

going to three museums in a row

the perfect spot

starlit beaches

being addicted to systematically popping
the bubbles of packing material

Imagine that!

herringbone twill pants

adjusting the sugar/cream level of your
coffee and catching the waitress
before she pours more in

pens with clocks on them

the night smell, feel, and wonder of
October

glazed pears

stuffing a phone booth with people

skewered dinner on the grill

swimming with dolphins

making a wish list and then taking action
so the wishes may come true

sturdy plastic plates, knockabout cutlery,
simple gingham napkins, and an old
blanket to spread on the ground

remembering to take the shampoo into
the shower

appearing on your favorite late-night talk
show

bring-a-friend parties

Kriss Kringle

white wicker furniture contrasting with
a patterned brick floor, jungle plants,
and a fountain

sleuthing with Nancy Drew through all the
    great series' books
taking Christmas cookies to friends
empty bottles when you need them
scrubbed and oiled baked potatoes, not
    cooked in foil
regional, semi-state, and state baseball
    championships
"California Dreamin'" by the Mamas and
    the Papas
pouring milk into a cereal bowl and
    knowing to stop when the edge starts
    to move
abstract art
taking advantage of walking weather
the flashy, robust season of fall
cheese and crackers served from atop an
    old potbellied stove
the persistence of dandelions
Swiss steak sandwich with butter and salt
tyrology, a set of instructions for
    beginners
fields of tall yellow flax stalks
something a child taught you
plate-size cinnamon buns
pizza, stamp, poker table, and gumball
    jigsaw puzzles
Memorial Day parties
being offered free HBO or other premium
    channels

people who know exactly where they're
    going
the sweet crunch of corn on the cob
getting your eyeglasses adjusted perfectly
laying in a supply of paper plates and
    taking a week's vacation from
    dishwashing
tiny graph-paper checks
a high-yield savings account
a quiet observer
peach melba with whipped cream
the flavor and ambience of the
    Maine woods
puffy sleeves
walking through fresh snow and listening
    to it crunch
Dictionary Day, October 16
the fun activity you saved for the end
    of the day
the upward flight of skyscrapers
an illuminating encounter
tester beds
a great cat named Sidney
an echo
crème de menthe (mint) parfaits
pancake tossing
honesty being so delightfully, pink-
    cheekedly seductive
someone who looks right at your eyes and
    smiles a huge, sweet smile

fresh and tangy lime
noticing how dirty your windows are and
    knowing that winter is almost over
spaghetti sauce
making full use of a season pass
marble sinks
toast points
linden trees
in the autumn, ravines aglow with the
    fiery brilliance of sugar maple and
    witch hazel
tic-tac-toe in the dirt
a gentleman and a scholar
sleeves pushed up for hard work or eating
apple and sweet-potato puree, served with
    pork or chicken or at breakfast with
    sausage or bacon
putting food by
moving from the needlings of nervous
    energy to a deeper level of stillness
chipmunks garnering grass seed and
    lining nests with thistledown
a baseball game going into extra innings
reusing an old bridesmaid's dress
good-bye to "the new math"
fire escapes slashing down sides of
    buildings like wrought-iron lightning
scoffing at superstitions
bleached, ultrafaded blue jeans
V-8 with lemon

hot chocolate and big marshmallows after
　　being outside in the cold
seeing 200 sails or hot-air balloons of
　　different colors
a porch full of jack-o'-lanterns
woven baskets
all-night jam sessions
cats and blowing leaves
unusual artichoke plates
small packages wrapped with foil papers,
　　bits of calico, embroidered ribbons,
　　lace, and tiny flowers
the Mach band that runs along the edge of
　　the sky and touches the ridgeline just
　　after sunset
writing labels to record a preserve's fruit
　　and birth date
a rasher of bacon done to a turn
handcuff-size onion rings
barrettes
dancing with a lover to 1950s music
bays and marinas jammed with boats
a quiet, intelligent game that encourages
　　people to think
inserting tabs
the exploration of Africa
chocolate-dipped graham crackers
bouquets of old-fashioned country flowers
a barn home or studio
riding the wind

the preposterous rituals that people resort
    to to get rid of hiccups
sailing picnics
Old Town, Wells Street, Chicago
celebrating togetherness
art classes
apple tarts
the cold coming and knitting a film of ice
bangs that finally grow out
BLTs at the corner coffee shop
kiln-dried oak
making words from Alpha-Bits cereal
the tradition of wedding spoons
being an archaeologist in your own
    backyard
traditional chants sung at the butter
    churner
the lure of the uncertain
playing kick-the-can
Sweetest Day, the autumn Valentine's Day,
    third Saturday in October
long, flat berry baskets
caramelizing onions
a wool gabardine Baltic cap with
    commander's scrambled-egg visor
marriage certificates
outdoor chaises
bird safaris
a small fragrant disk of sausage
walking a sandbar

barns sweet with hay and leather
the commonest words: *the, of, and, to, a,*
    in, that, is, I, it, for, as
Dijon mustard and freshly ground pepper
    to add spice
fabric patterns: check, cord, dapple,
    diamond, dot, floral, geometric,
    herringbone, pincheck, plaid,
    polychromatic, print, rib, solid,
    speckle, stripe, swirl, windowpane
pilots in uniform
purse atomizers
gumbos and jambalayas
low-bush blueberries
Cobb salad with Gorgonzola dressing
when your fingertips have shriveled like
    prunes and you're clean enough to
    put on fresh pajamas
white china drawer pulls
apple squares dipped in cream cheese
your favorite kind of clothes hanger
indirect lighting
the Boston Children's Museum
intellectual rigor
matryoshka, nesting dolls in a doll
the spicy odor of lasagna
well-coordinated charm
many surprises coming in one day
gizmos
winning acclaim

Walt Whitman's *Leaves of Grass*

Bibb lettuce

alarm clocks

greeting cards that "say" something

the energy to squeeze some juice, grind some coffee, and stir up a batch of muffins

little things

cream or half-and-half?

the Andy Warhol "famous for 15 minutes" philosophy

blankets: baby, cotton, down, electric, horse, military, thermal, woolen

polished ash or walnut wood

long walks across the frozen lake to the post office

flickering lights with shimmering reflections

a trout pond

watching it snow

three-gallon ice-cream tubs

bathing-suit season

singing along with a Beatles song

reading four dictionary pages a day

note-taking in college

scenic, sandy, salubrious Cape Ann

words pertaining to the nose: sneer, sneeze, snicker, sniff, sniffle, snipe, snivel, snob, snoop, snoot, snooty, snore, snort, snout, snub, snuff, snuffle

living in a 200-year-old house

pitching tents, setting the campfire blazing, and serving spaghetti with meatballs and tossed salad

the *Veronica Mars* crowdfunded movie

red Ferraris

1960s music

Vermont's atmosphere

chopping veggies with a mezzaluna

Shari Lewis and Lamb Chop the sock puppet

daring to write on the lines as well as in between them

cicadas' shrill songs

ethnic grocery shops

the sounds of geese high overhead

the softness of a kitten's feet, like raspberries held in the hand

a shade that lets in just the right amount of light

salmon color, an orange-pink

cozy robes, morning newspapers, chocolates on the pillows, milk and cookies at bedtime, and coffee 24 hours a day

TV show recaps/synopses

child-drawn maps of imaginative worlds

cashing in your chips

the silence of close friendship

smile lines

accidental meetings
young robins trailing their mothers
    on a search for worms
Mozart piano concertos
strapless bras
forest walking
exclaiming, "Works for me!"
kids keeping you moving
Central American bananas
a 4-foot Christmas tree
dolman sleeves
sofa beds
selling subscriptions
how maps are made from satellite photos
small snowmen with twigs for arms
flat, smooth, cool sand,
    just out of reach
    of the incoming tide
a 20-hour workweek
starting an herb garden
carrots growing deep
the snort of a nose-blower
The Wizard of Oz (movie)
putting on heavy ski socks and a good
    warm bathrobe
a very soft, old-fashioned teddy bear with
    plaid paws, ears, and ribbon
staring off into space
the light of two lamps mingling
getting tickets to a play

writers' houses strewn with "tools of the
   trade"
old calfskin wallets
mountain-climbing over molehills
buying some lacy underwear and wearing
   it for everyday
a zillion breezy notions
buttery suede slippers
remembering coed night at the health club
television broadcasts from space satellites
sleep
the fragrance of cookies baking
chicken pot pie
steak-bite appetizers
seeing the moon rise
an outdoor cat tent
alpine trails above the timberline
a tailgate picnic before the kickoff
old Bible racks hooked on a cabinet to
   hold cookbooks
a bright red maraschino cherry atop
   a snow-capped whipped cream
   mountain
white doves restlessly circling a château
soup du jour
discovering that there is no real difference
   in the various cycles of your washing
   machine
being a playground leader
paint rollers

watching out for traffic, holding hands,
    and sticking together
the rare pileated woodpecker
butcher coats
a candlelight parade or procession
unconventional tablecloths: country quilt,
    painter's dropcloth, unfolded road
    map, sheet of butcher's paper, tartan
    wool blanket, festive rag rug
not taking your computer's health for
    granted
winter, a time to emulate nature
memories of Hostess Twinkies
green candles sitting on a bed of leaves
the total points in a winning dart game = 0
a screened-in gazebo
a 20-question marathon in the car
baby dandelions
night music
Elmer's Glue-All
letting color predominate
exploring, taking chances, being
    adventurous and spontaneous
Crenshaw melon
wilderness jeep safaris
the field hockey team in college
desk cubbyholes
cheese samples
a wire Easter-egg dipper
mustache wax

recharging with a catnap
a wife and a husband as best friends
meatballs in onion gravy or barbecue
    sauce
comfy chairs in large bookstores
the Sunday paper on the back porch with
    a hot beverage
children who behave in restaurants
little graces
"S" pothooks
a tall octagonal aquarium
experiences and interactions with the
    world through art, intellect, and/or
    emotional ties
plants you can take care of
calling ahead to order your favorite potato
    salad
letting go of inhibitions without need of
    excuse
buying fresh flowers
counting the miles
an evening of zero productivity
gnomes, leprechauns, and trolls guarding
    treasure
a reading nook
simple syrup
LaPorte, Indiana
an area that is happily underdeveloped
    and underpopulated
city britches

when you pour soda and the fizz shoots
    right to the brim, you expect it to
    overflow, but it slowly drops down
New Mexico: mesas, canyons, caverns,
    pueblos, Taos
blue pencils
strawberries and powdered sugar
packing a flask of spiked coffee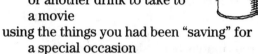
    or another drink to take to
    a movie
using the things you had been "saving" for
    a special occasion
spareribs cooked in pineapple juice,
    garden corn on the cob dripping with
    butter, and fluffy mashed potatoes
    with no lumps
wading knee-deep in fallen leaves
the cheery glow of a crackling fireplace
tin-lined copper pans
gooseneck floor lamps
when the dog brings the paper and there's
    not a hole in the middle
straw fedoras
narrow columns of type, meant to be read
    quickly
a contemplative corner of your own
being booted, mufflered, and storm-
    coated
shells collected from the beach with
    single orchids growing out of them

aging a stew or soup
lengths of knotty pine for a paneled effect
the sloshing of soft bristles around a
soapy mug
singing waiters and waitresses
aglets: shoelace tips
seeing a rainbow
sipping fun down to the last drop
Easter basket treats
when someone throws you a curve and
you roll with it
red ribbons tied in bows around tree
limbs
nondairy cream
seeing interesting people in an elevator
asking for a booth at the restaurant
a dollar-store tchotchke
a scarecrow that you think is working
garbanzo and cannellini beans
a band concert
turning your pillow over and over, seeking
a cool spot
parsley-butter patties on steak
satiny shirts
a Greek picnic: bread, feta cheese, salad,
and wine
colorful shopping bags loaded to the brim
people who just by their presence warm
your heart
the regular harbor contingent of mallards

a cat attacking a toy or wrapping paper

adopting a parakeet and teaching it to talk

what paintings do after-hours in a
    museum

the unmistakable message of love

boneless prime-graded, dry-aged strip
    steak in a black mantle of char

boys' bikes

getting home, turning off the cell phone,
    turning on the radio, and hopping into
    a scent-filled tub for one hour

trying to figure out the theme of a
    conversation in a foreign language

LinkedIn and networking on it

appetite-whetting exercise

thinking good thoughts

shining, smiling, sweetly peanut-buttered
    faces

paper cups of cinnamon-flavored
    applesauce

a troop of kangaroos

writing down all the different roles you
    play

the tickling sensation of face painting

red-carpet treatment

prodigal sons

the segments of the crustacean body

when the whole school is assembled
    in the auditorium to watch a space
    launch

a cascade of foliage
the common people: hoi polloi
"Next window, please" signs
speaking kindly
pinning your hat on
philosophies on posters
going to an outdoor café
spray-on peroxide hair lightener
a beloved pair of cushy shoes
birthday wishes that come true
absorption of information
gourmet provisions for a weeklong
    adventure
the unpredictableness of life
signs on old jalopies
open-air cinemas
experimenting with color
cozy rooms with pretty details
the dignified face of a woman well into
    her 80s
fresh air after a stuffy room
lingering over coffee and buttered muffins
small evergreen hedges
dimmers for lights
things that are quiet and old and simple
    and ordinary and very real
paper quilling
listening to chickadees
horn-rimmed glasses
the inn's boat launch

a bird feeder hanging outside a sunroom
     window
slicing a fruit into a continuous helix
a new bedspread
apple blossoms
morning prayer
Quonset (or Nissen) huts
tubs of Pepsi bottles and ice
survival manuals
the tangerine flash of Baltimore orioles
a real person answering the phone
planning an audition for a community play
someone who likes Brussels sprouts
the soul-stirring sound of rain on the roof
tagless T-shirts
having a field day
peanut butter and cranberry sauce
     sandwiches
bleached or stenciled floors
potato and cheese blintzes as large as toss
     pillows
the "lucky" bay leaf if it ends up in your
     portion
old country inns to get lost in
seedless oranges
story hour
collapsing on the bed and cuddling
smells of grilling meat and veggies filling
     the warm air
bridle paths

a soul mate
Christmas shopping online
heirloom family pictures
Jack and Jill
the pure promise of dawn
fads you've embraced
quiet times
soothing your temper
bald lights
cooking on a real fire
the manual alphabet
crayons that don't go through the wash
Quincy Market, Boston
equinoxes and solstices
ice-cold melon
the damask whorls of a napkin
rope hammocks
a tool organizer bucket from Duluth
    Trading
painting only the ceiling
extra kisses
dogs that guzzle from a dish,
    shed profusely, nap on the
    living room sofa, and sleep on
    a family member's bed
weekend pants
high chairs
solar heating
color-coordinated undies
listening to a child

a spinning potter's wheel
breakfast at the bird feeder
jumping on a pogo stick or walking
     on stilts
beachfront vacations
cross-country trekkers
reading slang dictionaries for chuckles
tableside steak Diane and Caesar salad
large-button calculators
welcoming the new person at school
a pet, hot chocolate, and wearing your
     flannel pjs in bed
soapstone boxes
frosty chains and pom-poms on a
     Christmas tree
getting really good meat from the butcher
whizzing down hills with wind on your
     face and sun on your back
shirts trimmed with ribbon
seeing America by bicycle
George Gershwin, composer
the day when the air-conditioning can be
     turned off
life moving in mysterious ways
yellow colonial glassware
tufted-leather banquettes
the Kia Soul (car)
frozen ice on a stick
an asterisk with no corresponding
     footnote

a miniature trampoline
classic Seville and coarse-cut orange
     marmalades
ham-filled crepes and lots of good cream
     sauce
listening to Mozart and feeling like tulips,
     warm breezes, boats on the lake, and
     sailor hats
harmless flirting
Japanese lanterns strung between trees,
     gently lighting the lawn
watching Emeril Lagasse cook
the Bluebird of Happiness
lover's-knot doormats
McDonald's Egg McMuffins
baking a variety of breads and serving
     them hot with a crock of butter
autumn feasts
an unexpected letter
sticky fingers after eating cotton candy
jet streams
curling up in bed on a Sunday afternoon,
     then reading a book until dawn
election returns
a hands-free phone
Moon: the night light of Earth
family resemblances
the first college weekend
bird nerds
lemon zest strippers

crème brûlée
mobiles moving gently
childhood friendships
track shorts
lamb's wool and angora
corn silk
Botts' dots
lemon balm
short explanations
zippers of sunbeams seaming up their
    light
pull-up diapers for babies
the calm of the day after Christmas
sweet-and-sour chicken
your oldest living relative
newborn puppies with trip-over ears
splendid "dunkers" with coffee
colorful surprises
throwing a football in the backyard
having a heart-to-heart with Dad or Mom
new potatoes steamed in their jackets,
    sweet and moist, with a light spicing
    of salt and herbs
webbed army-type belts
bright wallpaper and white ceilings
pastel colors
diamond mines
quilted kitchen appliance covers
chubby cows chewing contentedly on
    the grass

inch-thick, golden brown French toast
Oxford shirt collars being sexy
samovars, urns with a spigot
deviled eggs
phantasmagoria
potatoes and onions fried with hot spice
finger bowls and turn-down service
antifreeze
animal sounds
having the cleanest car in town
Dutch scenes on the ends
    of demitasse spoons
apple cider
Paris Match (magazine)
software for learning a foreign
    language
yawning being good for you
a space suit
houseboats
a small candle glowing in a wineglass
knowing it's almost spring when people
    are starting to panic about income
    taxes
tucking a paperback into a friend's purse
    or putting a tiny plant on his or her
    windowsill
popular opinion
talking calmly about problems
the popularity of the mango
the humor in static cling

dressing business casual
floor-to-ceiling windows
patio carts
light verse
smiling at someone who never smiles at you
hothouse tulips
European square pillows
French-vanilla sheets
white carved statues
constructing an ontology
stand-up desks
carrot-and-raisin slaw
deep-sheared terry cloth
It's a Wonderful Life, A Christmas Carol,
    and *Miracle on 34th Street* (movies)
love of books
vacationing on a farm in Denmark
medieval market squares
being the only one awake in the morning
tiptoeing into a room
relying on the cat to remove crumbs
    from the floor
bedtime snacks
cruising on a longboard
having an advantage over every other
ambidexterity
being unable to tell a lie
putting yourself in the server's place
dark wood floors warmed by Oriental,
    kilim, or needlepoint rugs

early morning eateries
nubby cotton
a sleek or tiny cell phone
using the soupspoons
tennis on public courts
bookcases in kitchens
making your own dough ornaments
honoring a longstanding agreement
rooting for the underdog
tweaking
women who look like they stepped out of
    a page in a French fashion magazine
birch trees, flashing and fluttering
the exquisite sweetness of the air above
    snow
literary guilds
double dares
pie wedges
butter-making
an inflated glitzy metallic balloon
Mattel toys
steam rooms
the philosophy of Socrates
sentiment and a sense of history
marinated vegetables
frogs in unexpected places
poetry accompanied by percussion
sweet potatoes ripening in the sun
vacation dates
tiny picturesque harbors

sizzling steak fajitas
eating breakfast on your front stoop
summer cardigans
savory food
notebooks that open flat
automobile running boards
the six ways a batter can get on base
    without getting a hit
the original Equal Rights Amendment's
    ideals
fresh asparagus soup garnished with
    slivers of ham
not watching the CNN or MSNBC crawl
pressed-glass candlesticks
barefoot beachcombing
honey-colored paneling and flooring
camel, spice, and whiskey colors
the fried dough wagon at the fair or
    flea market
Sunday rides in the country
moonlight talks
honeysuckle reaching upward for light
a thumbs-up
snow picnics
emoticons
dinner at noon
encouraging someone to take up a hobby
A&W root beer
actions speaking louder than words
parti-colored things

the ancient city of Petra
trees twinkling with ice
a European side street
Milano, Lido, and Brussels cookies
glints of firelight throughout a room
embroidering folkloric flowers with
    picoted icing
mirrors that distort you
island exploring
squirrels gathering nuts early
cobblers' aprons
a child who understands "no"
debating half in jest
herb-lined pathways where one pauses
    to savor the smells
soft, worn jeans
table linens
the ability and the need to be creative
the gentle dip of a paddle
flower seeds
multicolored rag rugs
ankle-tied espadrilles
scones and honey and marmalade
mini-cliffhangers
the perfect detective story
flip-down airplane trays
examining the words preceding or
    following the one you looked up in a
    dictionary or thesaurus
cloudy days and sunny thoughts

vinegar to soothe a sunburn
saucerlike eyes
toy doctor/nurse kits
spending a night in an igloo
footed bathtubs
relaxed neck muscles
eating three slices of pizza and the
      next morning finding you're
      a pound lighter
hauling out photo albums dating back to
      high school
air-traffic controllers
bumper pool
code names
the tiny bags for hardware (screws, etc.)
      they use at Ace Hardware stores
a bravely patient tree leaning leafless in
      the wind
lucrative seasonal employment
sit-up pillows for the bed
scrub brushes
country roadsides sweet with clover
Iowa City, Iowa
being the best putt-putter around
revolving doors
ages and eras of history
reminiscing while listening to Frank
      Sinatra
hunches
being happily bushwhacked

football-watching snacks
not sulking
sailor collars and shirts
South Carolina: stately
     gardens, white-pillared
     homes, cotton, sweet jasmine
carrying a spare tire
Slo-Poke, 3 Musketeers, Nestlé Crunch,
     Chunky, Kit Kat, Heath, and Skor
     (candy bars)
ground beef casserole (otherwise known
     as Hamburger Surprise)
sundae dishes
berry-picking excursions
amicable divorce
tumbling down a meadow's hill
kitchen sinks
the patter of dozens of feet on pavement
scraping snow and ice off the car
mind-over-matter philosophy
summer league baseball and softball
toilet kits
Pennsylvania: coal, liberty, midpoint of 13
     colonies, laurel, mountains, steel
passing a federal exam
bacon tasting like salt, honey, brown
     sugar, or maple syrup—or like
     hickory, mahogany, apple wood, or
     oak smoke
Georgia peaches

cool beans
Châteaubriand for two
Plato and Aristotle, philosophers
onion soup mix and sour cream dip
tae kwon do practice
steaks with mushroom sauce, peeled
    baked potatoes, and salad
getting out of class to set up for school
    dances in the gymnasium
seed money
the setting sun creating great red and
    orange streaks over the snowy hills
shoveling the sidewalk
wedding invitation charms
monumental beauty that you would hit
    the brakes for
hot chocolate sauce of a deep, cocoa-like
    strength
beach volleyball
picking handfuls of purple violets,
    dogtooth violets, and anemones
"the big cheese" and "the second banana"
Edward Bear: Winnie-the-Pooh's real
    name
the ablative tense
the squeak of Styrofoam picnic chests
an after-dark ramble to search for fireflies
    and listen for night sounds
deadbolts
marveling at fairy-tale trees iced in snow

attending to your own business and never
     trusting it to another
riding stables
wooden fences bordered by colorful
     peonies
chimney tops puffing
discovering the mystery buttons' uses on
     a remote control
paisley scarves from the Provence region
     of France
being tapped as someone walks by
the window sticker on your new car
roadside tables piled high with fresh eggs
     and produce
hanging up clothes in color order
aluminum, extracted from bauxite, the
     most plentiful metal in the Earth's
     crust
Venetian blinds between two windows,
     found in Europe
snack sessions
the name "Holly Beth"
professional organizers
a timid tiger
soft maples in the swamp
starting a garden on the windowsill
pachyderms
lemon-sesame sauce for grilled vegetables
a crushed oyster-shell path
a deep, elegant, or beautiful explanation

hearing, "Who loves you, baby?"
the rattle of an old truck
Turkish taffy
self-sufficiency, self-respect, efficiency,
and the discipline of hard work
participating in karaoke night
maintaining a continuous state of
thanksgiving
delis with short waiting lines
a trip to the encyclopedia
cream of leek and potato soup
meat pounders
walking bravely on ice
dimples
generous words toward others
owning a house
microwave ovens
cherry tomatoes stuffed with deviled ham
Saturday night with Garrison Keillor and
A Prairie Home Companion on NPR
dance marathons
Je reviens, meaning "I will return"
sets of artists' colors
getting the teacher you wanted
a three-chair barbershop with shelves of
colorful shaving mugs
Santa's kitchen
nonprofit organizations
sun burning off the morning fog
brick-and-board shelving

word-a-day calendars
smelling the bakery on your street
temptations
curling up in a ball
spring bazaars
a room decorated for fall with pumpkins
and Indian corn
power players
knackwurst, bratwurst, Italian sausage,
and chorizo
calling a worker after you received
exceptional service, just to say
"Thank you"
flatscreen electronics
fillets and chops merrily sizzling away
honey mustard sauce
crackle in the fall air
cottage cheese and fruit
whale-watching cruises
1-2-3-BUZZ game
not waiting too long
Marilyn Monroe, actress
the old Danish custom of tying a knot
at a wedding
brooding about the meaning of life
dance halls
candles glowing in the entryway
white spring flowers, green and white
Chinese vegetables, and bottles of
wine in crushed ice

moist gingerbread and cranberry nut bread

come-as-you-are parties

the joy of discovering a second layer of chocolates underneath the first

newer late-night talk show hosts like Jimmy Fallon, Conan O'Brien, and Stephen Colbert following in the footsteps of their predecessors

frosty shades

the morning waitress

a variety of watercolor palettes

hobby shops

mousse cups

magazines that you've read for decades

roadside displays of wild aster and fringed gentian

nanoscience: the study of manipulating materials on an atomic or a molecular scale

making decisions to benefit more than just yourself

a wienie roast in the woods with logs as seats, 7UP, and barbecue chips

pencil-striped clothing

your best bib and tucker

protected inventions

Scotch pine trees

praising your teammates

the fireplace as a combination of
sentiment, emotion, and vague
memories
want-to, have-to, ought-to feelings
small pieces of toilet paper applied to
shaving wounds
Despicable Me (movie) minions
a library step for high-up bookshelves
meringues that melt in the mouth
Friday, otherwise known as "weekend eve"
bookmobiles
new friends to help us stay young
Pollyanna's collection of prisms
doubling the temperature and adding 30
to convert Celsius to Fahrenheit
conflicts with an umbrella on a windy day
loop buttoning
alley cats
the all-American cranberry
old wicker chairs with floral fabric-
covered seats
the electric touching of fingertips
Danish potatoes
the thrill of fresh starts and unimagined
adventures you feel when you buy a
new journal or notebook
a sense of serenity
giving thanks for what you have
living alone
responsible, professional reporters

self-taught woodworkers
upward mobility
one of those "Who knew?" places
grand slams
anniversary dinners
using any item within reach to help grab
  the remote control so you don't have
  to move
buying a set of postcards at a museum to
  bring the museum home with you
hot lobster rolls with melted butter
deep leather couches
horoscope junkies
anything 'n' cream ice cream
watching cats "meditate"
press secretaries
tooth fairies
inspecting big caldrons bubbling with
  apple butter
cold vegetable salads
using the vacation time you have
  accumulated
knowing that someone somewhere
  understands you
learning a new job skill
crib sets
letting kids be kids
Reuters and the Associated Press
colors intense against pale sand
Mrs. Butterworth's syrup bottles

bamboo cutting boards
phone-answering services
tearoom food
slatted doors
lemon butter pats and mint on peas
monogrammed jewelry
someone to carry heavy things for you
airy, Frenchified cakes and pastries,
     extremely pretty, creamy, and rich
renting a barge for a special event
oak moss, balsams, leaves, woods
making a package store run
the ability to adapt to almost any situation
     and to make do with whatever is at
     hand to reach a goal
PTA potluck dinners
going to bed before you get sleepy
crisp blue-and-white plaid and rich yellow
     upholstery adding to natural wood
     and brick tones
sweatpant drawstrings that don't retreat
electric heating pads
fire engines
paperback guidebooks
the Tao of homemaking
composing songs
being devoted to something outside
     yourself
dragging out an old washtub, sitting under
     a tree, and tipping the hose in

kitchen work islands
relaxing to the creak of an arthritic rocker
bleached floors, white fabrics, and greenery
strawberries in a pineapple boat
bus terminals
making a movie
classically cut trousers with pocket
    on seam, straight leg, cuffed
giant slices of slightly caramelized
    apple on pastry
butterscotch blondies
potato skins with bacon, cheese,
    chives, and sour cream
three-point basketball shots made at
    the buzzer
a river of hippos
dinghy boats
antique trunks
being here, now
taking a walk in the woods with a field
    guide to identify trees, animals,
    and birds
making your own junk food at home
babies' name bracelets
secret formulas
sweatbands from the 1970s
ice-cream hugs and kisses
at least one "play break" each day
harp music floating in the air
a crab leg—very orange and fragile

the sidewalk sizzling your soles
two or more people unintentionally
    wearing the same thing
the whole world encompassed in a single
    leather-bound volume
packing twine
an electrician at the ready
frying eggs
faculty-student athletic contests for charity
sinking your teeth into fresh peaches,
    plums, watermelons, and apricots
gyro sandwiches and tzatziki sauce
the country, viewed through a curtain
    of warm summer rain, taking on
    exquisite watercolor tints from
    smoky blue to tarnished silver
a dresser in your closet
a roll of white paper, crayons, and
    imagination
framing the best Christmas cards
being motioned to come sit by someone
Henley-style Fair Isle sweaters
washing the car windows on the inside
the lovely names of algae like dulse,
    fucus, nostoc, pond scum, and wrack
floating flower candles
hearing a song that you haven't heard in
    a gazillion years and still knowing all
    the words
vanilla wafer crumb crust

tan and brown suedes and leathers
art techniques: airbrushing, collage,
     engraving, etching, finger painting, line
     drawing, melt-and-color, oil painting,
     pencil drawing, relief rubbing,
     scrimshaw, spatter painting, wash
     drawing, watercoloring, wood carving
brocaded robes
any refund
Amish buggies
summertime stripes
nonaerosol products
looking down on the world from the top
     of a Ferris wheel
early mornings
the pips on playing cards
Sunday morning at Home Depot
windshield wipers on eyeglasses
the nights beginning to draw in
the sayings of Lao-Tzu
clippity-clop, jingle-jingle sounds
cottage cheese and sugar
the habitats of waders and shorebirds
perky teapots
human ecology
tree-trimmed streets graced with
     antebellum mansions
a pastry board with patterns for rolling
     dough into a 10-inch pie
public relations

a keen curatorial eye for amassing a series
    of potentially unrelated artifacts and
    making sense of them
an early case of spring fever
eating cookies and milk in the car
belts with whale, geese, lobster, and
    yacht motifs
getting artsy-craftsy
achieving the "not-decorated" look
dry wood for kindling
corn poppers
new computers
the muffled clinking of silver from a tree-
    shaded patio
making something from magazine
    instructions
brimming glasses of ice-cold milk
father-and-son outings
thick slices of buttered sourdough toast
loud radios
a red tomato pincushion
shower massagers
half nelsons in wrestling
the flag flying
a happy snowman
lubricating your joints
lilacs "mauving" in the breeze
closing your eyes while listening to your
    favorite piece of music
having loved, lost, and loved again

group hugs

the duck-billed platypus

a lot of hooey

exchanging gifts on New Year's Day

attic sleuthing

good food for a cold afternoon: piping-
hot chocolate and crispy, home-fried
doughnuts

the zip of fly fishermen's rods

when all the company you've
got is silence

touring the Louisiana bayous

computer progress bars

a school's proud colors

the word *groovy*

tall candles

setting the table with cloth napkins and
napkin rings

Wassily Kandinsky and Paul Klee

sloshing around in waders

shy beginnings

watching with curious fascination

baby pictures, slides, and movies

paean, a song of praise or triumph

susurration, soft rustling or murmuring

something left over

singing groups

a riding lawn mower and the flat lawn
to go with it

toasting and buttering a little delicacy

community leadership
cookies made in stoneware molds
list poems
flapped pockets
when you put the key in the door and
    enter with awareness
school figures and free-skating
the study of wind resistance conducted
    by holding a cupped hand out the
    car window
apple crisp pie
a traveler coming upon canyons and
    hidden valleys, waterfalls, and
    freshwater springs
jokes at a testimonial dinner
the Dow Jones Industrial Average
long-stemmed carnations
banana peels
a salad of miniature marshmallows,
    pineapple chunks, pecans, and
    American cheese
a Sunday feast of pot roast or plump
    roasted chicken
the Olympics
a safe port in a storm
inhaling maximum amounts of sea air to
    stimulate the appetite
a shrug of the shoulder when things don't
    get done
a sampler at a brewery

not being hornswoggled

getting lost on purpose when you were little

the formation of English vocabulary from
    Latin and Greek

beating around the bush

rain sounding as though a thousand tiny
    flamenco dancers were rehearsing on
    the roof

tolerable temperatures

pumpkins lit to frighten witches

vegetable combinations

sea salt

classical music on the stereo

enjoying it while it lasts

saying a quick prayer

collecting colorful wine labels

battling for a rebound

endowing a scholarship

Chicago or Country Club ice cream:
    vanilla, orange sherbet, and coffee

taking dance lessons

the sneeze that tickles but never comes

one fantastic lover in college

delicate asparagus and artichokes, crisp
    lettuce, and new peas

ambling across fields with a sketchbook
    or camera

mounds of blueberry, apple, pumpkin, and
    date muffins

an intoxicating atmosphere

a perfectly chilled drink

decorating a bachelorette house exactly
  as you want

soda fountain treats

comic relief

scallop shells

fog hovering like a blanket above the
  ground, as if the world does not want
  to get out of bed

a solo drive down unexplored lanes

making college education inexpensive

cooperation

the ease of using a slow cooker

architects of international repute

your mind being at your command

a rousing choir practice

cast-aluminum skillets with wooden
  handles

using candles

laboratory research

zipper-front and button-fly jeans

Rhode Island: Newport, mansions,
  breakers, yachts, Block Island

Buddha nature: the true, immutable, and
  eternal nature of all beings

the end of summer traffic

a badger in the backyard

chicken roast with a light coating of
  thyme, tarragon, and onion powder

white-collar workers

a quick drop in temperature and then
    a gradual turn of the leaves
large etched-glass bowls for serving
    salads, fruits, ice cream
party plates
the hen coop
coffee barefoot (black)
boys in caps
hugging a teddy
fresh, chunky strawberry spread
the shower, where the acoustics are
    concert-perfect
large slices of tomatoes with goat cheese
    and balsamic vinegar
stapling papers for the study hall teacher
remembering what you have learned
Maine and Idaho potatoes
getting a sliver out
porch gliders
paying attention to how different kinds
    of music affect you
feeling really good, alive, aware, filled
    with a tingly sense of well-being
the energy points where needles are
    inserted for acupuncture
getting involved with people outside
    the usual circle of friends
the cool books sold at Urban Outfitters
looking on the bright side
baggy pants

stopping by the edge of a woodland and
finding dainty-flowered anemones
nodding brightly in the breeze
boned chicken breast in a sour-cream sauce
accented with sweet Hungarian paprika
clambering over rocks
satin Christmas balls
strong emotions
basket weaving
painting the apartment
invisible panty lines
recipes from old books
beautiful sand patterns
spending the day looking forward to an
evening home alone
white pizza with asparagus
bolts of calico fabric for sale
planting raspberries
grasping literal vs. figurative
casual partying
teriyaki sauce
the whimsy of kittens
a groomed athletic field
when sounds in the hotel don't wake you
fireflies blinking by
the light of Tuscany
overnighting in a yurt
a small music system in the kitchen
sugar syrup on grapefruit, apples, pears,
grapes, or blueberries

the blissfully splendid smell of mustard at
    the game
planning a hike
magnolia trees
gravy boats
bongo drums
old-fashioned door keys
a weekend afternoon taking photos
taco-flavored corn chips
chef's knives
having a good credit rating
prognostications
red lipstick
the whisper of an excited gathering
perusing the guest book at an inn
constantly changing stations on the
    car radio
ordering an Early Bird Special dinner
hair becoming blonder in summer
a yummy gourmet shop
the power of a touch, a smile, a kind
    word, a listening ear, an honest
    compliment, or the smallest act
    of caring
fine snow in the air
cargo pockets
forsythia buttering the roadsides
table legs that don't wobble
stocking fillers
using an alias

double-pack pinochle
brand-new sports facilities
red and Yukon new potatoes
waiting for the school bus
happily coping with cobblestones
encouraging the lost art of reading
a breath of fresh air
a rowboat with a motor
knowing when the generic product is just
    fine
grass's persistence
Worcestershire sauce
French playing cards
yellow and red roses for Valentine's Day
unique gift stores
peeling a hard-boiled egg and getting a big
    chunk of shell all at once
perfect couples
the uncurling of a fern
a group of kids with walkie-talkies in the
    woods
a pleasant song in your head
the buddy system
the spin of a football
a bachelor pad
fettuccine Alfredo
CEOs with ant farms on their desks
candle snuffers
the Grand Tetons
Chris Evert, tennis player

tasting sweet papaya and pineapple at a
    roadside stand
the pleasure of water
a time when you need extra love or
    attention and someone wants to give
    it unselfishly
old teddy bears
a gas cooktop
chimney pots
arts fanatics
kneading bread as therapy
dormer windows
the twang of a guitar
crayons in extremely obscure colors
going to sleep
progressive dinner parties
Nova Scotia
a small fishing village
firm mattresses
tortellini in pink cream sauce
thermos jugs of ice water
slowing down your speech
caramel apples
Naugahyde
oil wells being replaced by new energy
    technology
the essence of humor
the classic curves of old automobiles
a wicked jacks player
opening oysters

the Oxford comma
a basket of balloons
birthday celebrations
useful, preventive measures—the fruits of
    experience
going to a duty event, such as a political
    or volunteer meeting, and having it
    turn out to be fun
blond guys
a slippery firehouse pole
poring over a newspaper
Montpelier and Burlington, Vermont
extremely tiny pancakes formed from the
    batter that fell off the ladle
fry baskets dunked into hot oil
thinking in tune with someone
pet llamas
massive old breakfronts
finding a great answer to a science
    question
attending a concert after work
a barn full of books that cost 25¢ to $3 each
rugged clothes
having a dictionary by the bed
making a list of things that have been
    bugging you for a while
never being short on confidence
fishermen early in the morning
invisible ink
plain cottage cheese

a gnarled tree buffeted and timeworn,
    standing in stark silhouette
being able to hold a glass to your mouth
    by sheer lung power
pipsqueaks
realizing what a wonderful mate you have
music's affirmative character
thumb wrestling
L.L. Bean canvas totes
town halls
Tex-Mex food
a Chinese red lacquer coffee table
picking up your favorite cheeses
Rioja wine
sudden confrontation with a huge expanse
    of gentle hills and clusters of old trees
making fresh juice
a service counter in the kitchen
stubby tugboats
"I love it!"
exchanging news over tea
the screams of people riding roller
    coasters and splashing in the flume
bobbing markers for lobster pots
slices of watermelon with small seeds in
    them
Orthodox Easter's red eggs
long toothpicks
a born teacher
pumpkin soup in the fall

hot coals in the hearth for toasting toes

a Swedish flat whisk

an old-fashioned pole with a metal
grabber used for retrieving items
from high shelves

ripe cantaloupe

Victorian laces

mice outside

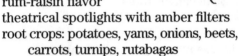

rum-raisin flavor

theatrical spotlights with amber filters

root crops: potatoes, yams, onions, beets,
carrots, turnips, rutabagas

slow sunsets

windshield wipers keeping time to the
music

lazy evenings

using less and less toilet paper as one
nears the end of the roll

custom cowboy boots, gingham dresses,
and broken-in hats

rushing rivers

a Swiss chalet dollhouse

floaty, filmy clothes

white: daisies, milfoil, Queen Anne's lace,
whitecaps on a windy sea

business suits

casual shoes

a bake sale with apple butter, dumplings,
sausage, scrapple, cider, and funnel
cakes

fraternity pins as a sign of intended future
     engagement
supernatural delights
gaslight-era frosted-glass ruffled bell
     lamps
sunglasses and shades
borrowing an RV
calculating tips using the sales tax
a room overlooking the lakeshore
wonderful serendipitous experiences
gourmet food clubs
cultural anthropology
conversational topics
a shady, babbling brook
candle-dipping demonstrations
marine paintings and prints
the folding process that allows Kleenexes
     to emerge from the box one at a time
tickets to the symphony
absence making the heart grow fonder
a ride home after dropping your car off to
     be serviced
being looked at
sharing things: toys, fun, giggles, secrets
what your wedding night was like
watching a wood turner make wooden
     bowls
the risk-reward ratio
baseball dugouts
customizing a template

the order of things
Mexican wedding cakes
basketball time buzzers
bouzouki music and blue, blue sea
cider made from bruised apples; apple
    juice from undamaged apples
playing a game of hopscotch with a
    neighbor
the history of phrase-making
having no noncompete clause
going up to the attic and finding 10 things
    to give or throw away
reflections of the seasons in constantly
    changing and inviting patterns of
    sights and sounds
fantod, one's nervous movements
going home
the purple, bell-like flowers of the false
    foxglove
Social Security number: first three
    numbers tell in what part of the
    country you were born; next two, a
    code for the year you were born; last
    four, your serial number
blue blazer, gray flannels, loafers, white
    shirt, and red-and-blue rep tie
solving problems
the need for imagination
gilt-edged picture frames
the phrase "not worth a red cent"

loving what you do
caller ID
overcoming distraction
sun sparkles
writing the phone number from the
     answering machine message correctly
     in just one listen
scrambled eggs with five cheeses
salt when you need it
smells of different gravies crowding the air
the NCAA's March Madness
learning to fly a plane
milking cows
the panic button
chenille
brand-new dominoes and checkers
a ghoulish coyote chorus
the Spot children's books
planning trips to country inns
pigeon heads bobbing
watching others play
bringing a blanket to sit on outside
     at lunch
feeding a hummingbird
summer dinner out in the garden
wooden spaghetti spoons
a really good hamburger
conchologists and their mollusks
the moon etching whimsical hieroglyphics
     on the snow beneath naked trees

simplicity and sophistication
clever columnists
the local lumberyard
full-skirt bathing suits
a pancake breakfast at town hall or the
    fire station
sitting on the deck of a sailboat
slumber parties or sleepovers
surrendering to "not knowing"
having a really good photograph taken
armfuls of spring flowers
an emotional refill
delivering compassion
when your story, poem, or article is
    published
spaghetti alla Bolognese
Lorna Doone cookies
rappelling cliffs
waiters in red jackets
daily joy breaks
modeling schools
cheese stores
Illinois: trains, Lake Michigan, wheat,
    stockyards, Chi-town
a June morning, the color of purest honey
love for nature
the very best tea, the very richest coffee,
    and the very thickest cream
candles of different heights on terra-cotta
    saucers

making simple wooden toys
inn and B&B cookbooks
scarlet ribbons
icy clear water
having a heart
fluffy sweet potatoes
houses clustered like barnacles
    on the hills
a sewing nook
putting a flower on someone's pillow
times when you can see, but not be seen
plastic colored Easter eggs that split
serene statues of Buddha
a complete paradox
taking someone to work
places where you need a Tundra Buggy
    or Sno-Cat
IMAX movies
traveling on a freighter
creative photography
hanging a favorite quilt on the living room
    wall behind the sofa
designing advertisements
hours of climbing trees
fending off a pushy salesperson
salads dressed and tossed at the table
bacon, eggs, sausage, coffee, cereal,
    pitchers of milk, apple butter, two kinds
    of fresh rolls, and gallons of juice
keeping busy at your highest natural level

Goldilocks and the Three Bears

quixotic: foolishly romantic, extravagantly
    chivalrous

slingback espadrilles

wooden book stands for large dictionaries

sweeps of white beach that surround the
    ocean's edge

an oversize mohair sweater and new
    tapestry flats

clear-blue creek waters

Daddy smoking his pipe in the family room

walking between the raindrops

finding a TV series to binge-watch over
    the holidays

homemade egg noodles

a steam explosion of corn kernels

self-serve anything

love that lasts and lasts

a sitz bath

nubby wools in solids and tweeds,
    abundant flannels, gabardines,
    camel's hair, cashmere, alpaca

an irresistible party mood

adjustable chamber candlesticks

anyone who knows what trigonometry is

a romantic holiday with one special person

the reporter on the police beat

a chocolate stash

cold cucumber soup, made hot, then chilled

horse prints and hunting scenes

finding a genuine arrowhead
perfect summer parties
a torchlit ski down the slopes
patterned silk ribbons
butternut squash bisque with apples
sleepy dogs
primitive reproduction paintings
compulsive crossword-puzzle doers
your all-time favorite coworker
Coca-Cola dispensers
seeing the world as it is
plain lo mein
gardens planted with cold-weather crops:
    turnips, broccoli, cauliflower, and peas
waffles topped with berries and peaches,
    nectarines, apricots, or bananas
coffee beans and a grinder
grocery bags with handles
police and firemen's badges
a gold tooth replaced by a crown
wine-dark sea
the way it felt to hit typewriter keys
a Swedish country inn set well off the
    main road
the domino theory
using a shoe to hammer a nail into a wall
telephone and television cables attached
    to the house, swinging and creaking
    in the wind
moderation

chamber music
pretty floral-patterned plates
judo belts
the Seven Dwarfs: Bashful, Doc, Dopey,
     Grumpy, Happy, Sleepy, Sneezy
when the one stock you own skyrockets
knowing what a quart is
filling out a "How was the service?" card
reference books
driving safely through a caution light
the prospect of teleporting
being a chaperone for the trip to the
     natural history museum
recovering workaholics
small bells hung from pagoda roofs
English farmhouse Cheddar cheese
making a wish on a ladybug
liquid diets
yellows, oranges, and rusty greens of the
     hickories, sumac, and beeches
Rolex-watch copycats
a night breeze gently nudging the
     sailboats
an old-fashioned brass telephone with
     separate earpiece
letting your hair dry in the sun
packing weeks ahead of schedule
a picnic in an orchard
andirons and fireplaces
a healthy alliance

dream yoga, sleep learning, lucid dreaming
powder-blue icebergs
koala bears
making a new bed in the spring
decorated Christmas trees
a baggy-eyed baker on the night shift
shopping at a mall for two hours
beer gardens at fairs
earthenware butter tubs
the Noble Eightfold Path
florist boxes
keeping a smile on your face until the
    shutter clicks
plush parlor and dining cars
planning a hike, bike ride, or farmers'
    market visit
law-abiding citizens
drawing a self-portrait, a "selfie"
spice cabinets
watching kids ice-skate
shuffling through brittle leaves
park concerts
dark green upholstery
rearranging the house
more than 50 years of happy thoughts
social workers
something "selling like hotcakes"
at least one night having Lean Cuisine,
    Chinese food delivered, or delicacies
    picked up at a specialty store

birds' nests
a healthy sense of boundaries
tennis whites
mystery novels
summer houses
having someone to make you laugh when
     things are tough
sash windows that look out on the street
I-Ching predictions
"Old Kentucky Rain" by Elvis
educational puzzle maps of the United
     States
college rings
the great thing about humans being their
     ability to change
Chinese brocade diaries
summer-weight slacks
getting something fixed
appropriate behavior
pineapple-coconut flavor
an underground railroad
the condition of waking up with your
     pajamas turned 180 degrees
a class you want, offered at a time you
     can attend
hot, perfumed freshen-up towels
seeing the twinkling lights of
     town in the distance
a steak for two
butterscotch-colored straw hats

airmail routes

puzzles: acrostics, anagrams, charades, conundrums, crosswords, cryptograms, enigmas, mazes, palindromes, tongue twisters

cheering up a dreary desk

airtight alibis

rain-hatched mushrooms springing underfoot

avoiding people who make you feel guilty

Valentine's Day aluminum-wrapped shoe boxes for elementary school

screened-in porches with delightful views and breezes

a handy shoehorn

spending a weekend alone with the cat

getting your point across

a profound sense of well-being from an organized closet

dressing up for holidays as an adult

surprisingly good dining hall meals

fire embers seemingly endowed with a memory of the sun

an act of devotion

long, flowing skirts

peanuts and raisins mixed

the many names and shades of colors

never saying "reach out"

Sally Field as Gidget

fresh produce

the springy device attached to the back
of a door that prevents the doorknob
from marring the wall
a stable with a dozen island-bred palominos
waiters' serving stations
mail that is not all bills
rubber baby buggy bumpers (tongue
twister)
eschewing wrinkle creams
pinstriped baseball shirts
playing fair
a country mile
a quirkyalone, single and happy
climbing to a lookout point that offers
a sweeping panorama of the
countryside
chamois cloth
violin lessons
getting your sea legs
movie synopses
the far side of the moon
kindergartners on their first trip to the
library
the HOLLYWOOD sign
hot buttered rum in the bar of a country inn
winter woods whitening silently
garden benches
dots and dashes
track meets
love returned

previewing music before buying or
    downloading
the practice of Ayurveda
roads wide enough for only one car, with
    "meeting" places to wait
a wooden stepladder as plant stand
linking oneself with a great cause
being as cute as a bug
cutting tags off new clothes or pillows
curlicues
the wrapper of your favorite candy bar
savoring a quick "fix" from a novel or
    leafing through a travel magazine
    at lunch
playing holiday music
your values and intentions
a thermos of frozen fruit "slush"
an early evening under the covers
starting every day a little happier because
    you have the newspaper delivered
brunch in a dreamy garden setting
vending machines with good stuff
Oregon red raspberry, sun-ripened
    strawberry, black raspberry, wild
    Maine blueberry, Michigan red tart
    cherry preserves
buttered maple syrup
rain ponchos
going clamming
multicolored ski hats

nurturing your own spirit
varying your study spots
fast snowfalls
chocolate mints
being fresh from the shower in a big robe
　　with wet hair combed back
fall fashions
corn beginning to ripen
rare birds
farmhouses with silos waiting to be filled
perceiving the edges, negative spaces,
　　relationships and proportions, lights
　　and shadows, and the Gestalt (the
　　unique set of qualities, the thingness
　　of the thing)
tiramisu melting in your mouth
the baskets of a doughnut shop
being young at heart
a solo part
losing weight
attentiveness
being in the same boat as your best friend
going to Tiffany's and trying on rings
elopements
showing a child how much fun life can be
a lifestyle office, with places to meditate,
　　shoot hoops, take a nap
light timers set during your vacation
Mother Goose
brunettes

funny toes
a wire fence "crocheted" by snow
magic growing crystals for kids
sincerity
deliciously odorous onion rolls and an ice-
    cream scoop of creamy butter
the subtle shading and smell of a peach
being swift to hear, slow to speak
stage managers
Spirographs and Hot Wheels
moving into town from the suburbs
St. Joseph's aspirin for children
clouds of herbal essence
roaring fires
soap balls
the posts of a picket fence
comfort food
"Hold the bus!"
a wave at sea
leaf patterns
movie stars
rainbow Jell-O
French country pitchers
mint-frosted brownies
a thousand fantasies
wind circles in the sand from beach grass
the position of your head as you bite into
    a taco
the furniture on which the pets are
    allowed

brass upholstery nails studding a couch
    or desk
jubilant music booming from open windows
the first trip to look at colleges
social skills
pale radar screens flickering with activity
sending an unsigned card or Valentine to
    the person you have a crush on
the last piece of pie, saved for you
looking up words you don't know how to
    spell
a placid lake ruffled only by swans and
    other waterfowl
people who don't swear
cowslip leaves, cress, borage, chervil, vine
    tendrils, and pickled roots
a morning tea party: lighted fire, small
    clove-studded apples floating in hot
    cider, homemade toast with honey
    butter, and breakfast sausage cooked
    in maple syrup
before speaking, asking yourself: Is it
    true? Is it necessary? Is it kind?
working at a concession stand
a free lunch
rope weaving
a quiet, unspoiled island
collecting souvenirs: stones from the
    beach, an antique sewing box from a
    yard sale, a roll of snapshots

tape recorders
getting the gist of required reading from
  the first and last chapters and online
  reviews
newly paved or freshly graveled
  driveways
sexy music
telling a letter, "Have a good trip" as it
  goes in the mailbox
nonsmoking buildings and areas
paid-off loans
geysers bubbling up from the bowels of
  the earth
gateleg tables
sea breezes
the muscle that makes a smile, the
  risorius of Santorini
Shetland yarn
beach shacks in Hawaii
rushing brooks and dark, quiet forests
  beside the road
a cake baking
opening a box of old clothes and being
  enveloped by familiar scents
simple weeds blowing on a windy hill
healthful mountain air
washing the car while barefoot
roasting the corn, hurrying it to the table,
  buttering it well, salting judiciously
naval heroes

"Saturday's child works hard for a living."
zeitgeist
doing whatever you like best to relax you
taking fried chicken on an airplane
filing the taxes in March
diaper services
progressive jazz
Google Maps
the many ways that make a kid feel big
sinking into down pillows
backward letters used only on clubhouse
    doors
half-cooked sugar cookies
blueberry jam
cultivating the seeds of serenity
the golden blaze of April forsythia
charcoal-gray mirrors
knowing the definition when someone
    needs it
drag strips
coming from behind to win
looking back on the past with as much
    pleasure as you get from looking
    forward to the future
fancy combs for hair
travelogues
battening down the hatches
warm, dry socks
the cooing doves of morning
the studying of a menu

toilets flushing in E-flat
fried dough: puffy, flaky-crusted, steamy
inside, with a gentle, cakey chaw
the development of Buddhism
late roses
cracking open a new book
fashions for every season
cactus pears
jeep trips
George Carlin, comedian
your favorite type of New Year's Eve
the delicious smell of cooking food and the
hustle and bustle of the preparation
picnic baskets
winning a blue ribbon
hand-cranking a freezer of ice cream
talking intelligently, possibly brilliantly
dulcimer music
taking an hour a day for yourself
a goalkeeper's concentration
loose-leaf notebooks
private rituals
assorted-size canvases
educational software
Green Goddess salad dressing
pedal boating around small islands
singing "We Gather Together" on
Thanksgiving
echoes in a cave
large-boned people

when the no-see-ums aren't out

someone all mittened and scarved

mukluks: fur-trimmed animal skin boots

running your best time

the natural path that clings to the cliffs
high above the sea

corduroy wales rubbing together

classic steamer lounge chairs with teak,
brass, and marine varnish

your favorite camp song, candle scent, car
color, card game, cartoonist, casino
game, childhood pet, Christmas song,
color to wear, concession stand food

half-full, never half-empty

lemon-flavored portobello mushroom
sandwiches

blackened steak

Roadmaster tricycles

the "light/dark" knob on a toaster that
makes you think you're in control

Pennsylvania Dutch chicken-and-corn
soup

care labels on clothes

college yearbooks

sassafras

pictures of mixed vegetables

being rowdy

oven-baked potato sticks

things becoming clarified once you
nurture yourself

steaming teakettle water
old-fashioned alphabet blocks
eating apple pie and Cheddar cheese for
    breakfast
conch shells
rearranging the entire house in one day
Olympic hopefuls
finding things when you need them
the dust of everyday life
an African stone game called mancala
something that is heaven-sent
stretching muscles in the morning
modest cheerleader outfits
hundreds of tones of wool yarns side by
    side
shopping for new and used books
going to an oldie double feature at the art
    house
tall beeswax candles
things that don't cost a bundle
improving yourself
a splash pool for kids
fine damask linen napkins, hand-hemmed
    and graciously monogrammed
a dinner of favorite appetizers
falling stars after midnight
late-day lounging back at the hotel
rowing with the oars you have
rules of thumb
being as warm as toast

open-late shops
a restored nickelodeon
old-fashioned bridal gowns
an increase in your allowance
catching a butterfly in the palm of your
    hand and letting it go
secret drawers
being the guest of honor
gold ball earrings
English muffins, split and toasted hot with
    lots of butter and jam
whipping up a casserole
an office with a window
your favorite facial expression, family
    photo, farm animal, fast-food
    restaurant, font, football stadium,
    foreign film, frosting flavor
taking five
mechanical pencils
charcoal briquettes burning grayish-white
drowsy mornings
ice crystals so small, so light, that they
    float like mist and shimmer in a
    January sunrise
sherpas and muses
having your car warmed up by a loving
    soul before you go out on a cold
    winter morning
a wind farm
cool, rainy weekends for lots of reading

Occupant or Resident mail
being the sorority social chair
toddlers in firefighter hats
art journals
the determination of an understudy
visiting Alaska
canapé trays
red leotards
double-cut lamb chops
motorcyclists wearing helmets
observing tadpoles in a clear pond
penny-pitching games
when the rain stops and the sun comes
    out
S.W.A.K.B.A.L.W.S.: sealed with a kiss
    because a lick won't stick
being good at cutting your own hair
Americanisms and Canadianisms
the secretive quality of your neighborhood
    at night
white T-shirts
using a big word
studying in the library
sending home a menu, used train ticket,
    brochure from a hotel
a quotation from a favorite novel
croquet layouts
receding chins
less strenuous pleasures
blouses with Peter Pan collars

microwave/toaster/broiler in one
gold-threaded jewelry
growing food
the days of training bras
watching a thunderstorm
the catalog of ships in Homer's *Iliad*
light, fluffy ladyfingers
the declaration "We're Number 1!"
tying a dozen helium-filled balloons to a
    friend's car
a down-to-earth attitude
umbrella shade tables
Quaker Oats
finding your way through an office park
multicolored zafus, gomdens, and
    zabutons for meditation
a dry basement
the steadfast sun
heavy Romanian crystal
kicking your baggage to the airport counter
tiger-stripe cats
cheesecake topped with whipped cream
puddles percolating in the downpour
seeing your favorite teen movie again
International Morse Code
dogs wearing college mufflers
chiffon cake with ice-cream balls
recovering from culture shock
a veterinarian who makes house calls
watching the sun rise and set aboard ship

hand-blown posy vases
the tug of a trout stream pummeling at
     your waders
below a meringue, a lode of banana,
     butterscotch, lemon, chocolate, or
     coconut cream
fireflies flashing their taillights
multihued stones collected from a river
throngs of businessmen in suits
not making any excuses for 24 hours
an enthusiastic kiss
"Good morning, sweetums!"
riding bikes along a seawall promenade
your picture in the paper for something
     good
a smile you wear all over
casaba melon
Cambria natural stone countertops
arena football
going whole hog
the secret urge to expedite the person
     ahead of you through a revolving door
fried, roasted, and smoked drumsticks
     and wings of turkey, hot and cold
     crisp salads, and crusty pies
multigrain foods
sleepy times
buttercream candies
flower-decked balconies
giving yourself a mind massage

pizza stones for cooking in your oven
little boxes of breakfast cereal
secret messages
clear crystal
standing out in a crowd
same-day dry cleaning
a medicinal kiss on the forehead when
    you are under the weather
mineral oils
the kind of love summer nights were
    made for
Paul Newman and Robert Redford in
    Butch Cassidy and the Sundance Kid
a cluster of rock candy
yeast-raised doughnuts
"Hold the pickle, hold the lettuce"
    (advertising jingle)
schooners and sloops in the harbor
okra in stew
sea or woods patterns
acting goofy
where the buffalo roam
real mashed potatoes with melted butter
a cousin who is like a sibling
a backscratcher
the origins of holiday words
three kinds of people in the world: those
    who make things happen, those who
    allow things to happen, and those
    who don't care

a bonfire by the lake
Humptulips, Washington
taking off in an airplane
garden pots
Vermont granite
the land drawing a white sheet
    up to its chin

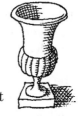

writing "Happy Birthday" on food
the sound of boats rocking in their berths
blood oranges for breakfast juice
being aware of wonder
Chicago's Field Museum of Natural History
bowls and baskets made out of bread dough
afternoons at garden fetes: flowered hats,
    tables laden with home produce,
    cakes, tempting offerings, milk for
    teas, and cream for scones
jam bubbling on the stove
helping each other grow
the little store on the corner
status quo institutions: piano lessons,
    ballet lessons, dancing school,
    French lessons, tennis lessons, sailing
    lessons, riding lessons, summer camp
imagining someone watching and
    admiring or desiring you
candied apples
on a weekend night, setting the alarm for
    2 a.m. to bake oatmeal cookies and
    read, write, or do whatever

honey and wheat germ
pick-your-own orchards
the gleaming cloud of your own breath,
    white and shimmering
the smell of toasted strawberry Pop-Tarts
Federal houses
taking three-day weekends in the summer
coincidences
wildlife in its natural habitat
a happily cloistered life
brown sweaters
square nails
plain or sugar ice-cream cones
root beer's foam, from
    yucca plant extract
picking fresh green beans
Florida oranges
sculpturing ribbons to ornament packages
    or hang on the tree
buying socks that fit
the sea's monumental indifference
Chip and Dale chipmunks
latte bowls
bowling balls
Indiana: basketball, covered bridges,
    steel, yellow poplars, popcorn,
    limestone caverns, Notre Dame's
    Fighting Irish
living in New England
quiet free hours to sit by a fire

dessert sauces: apple, blackberry,
blueberry, butterscotch, caramel,
cherry, cranberry, eggnog, mint,
orange fluff, peach, and strawberry
a summer hamlet where cottages and
picket fences crawl with wild roses
bread, still warm, in an unmarked plastic
bag tied with a snippet of wire
the toot of a train
getting a few more freckles
peacock throne chairs
a gift from the sea
innovative doorstops
letting someone have the last word
May baskets
the length of icicles
the truth, the whole truth, and nothing but
the truth
New Haven and Waterbury clocks
being silly and funny, serious and strict
a pantry with cubbies, bins, stacks, and
drawers
crashing a wedding with grace
two-year-olds without pacifiers
beautiful flower-decorated greeting cards
displayed in a basket
space pens that write on any surface,
upside down, forward, and backward
shoe tassels
red-tile roofs and rolling Pacific waves

someone understanding enough to hug
you soft and close when you cry, and
kiss away your tears
watching *Dead Poet's Society* (movie)
cognizance of the many hierarchies in the
world
cats sitting in the sun or by heating vents
a beauty shop appointment
fortune cookie pendants
chip-and-dip servers
visiting a formal garden on a sunny
afternoon
watching the rain fall
a new wax job on your car
"Thank you for not smoking" signs
stubby little drinking glasses
action photography
taper candles
racquetball courts
mud-thick Greek coffee
saying your piece
Gore-Tex and PrimaLoft
corn blades rustling, rabbits lying close,
the owl coursing the crisp meadow
on silent wings
hand-painted Chinese silk
parsley and watercress
days of ripened fruit
feeling a massive wave of relief washing
over you

flying in crosswinds

clean sheets

bare bricks and lantern lights

"Art is frozen Zen." (R.H. Blyth)

the aurora borealis

kindergarten drawings on the refrigerator

a baked bean supper on Saturday night
and a roasted chicken dinner at
Sunday noon

when designing a letterhead was as fancy
as one got

zoot suits

silly times

picking your own lobster from the
restaurant tank

Noah Webster's birthplace in West
Hartford, Connecticut

sewing scissors

the attuned eye/ear/mind finding "tongues
in trees, books in the running brooks,
sermons in stones"

a mixed bag

strange bugle sounds at basketball games

closing your eyes while riding on a
motorcycle

buy three, get one free

breezeless days

a couch potato weekend

a meadow, green with the freshness of
April

not traveling the world in search of what
    you have at home
a hot tub under the stars after a long day
    of backpacking
Russian salad dressing
meat cross-hatched with grill marks
rowdy times
amour
hooves on cobblestone
drawstring pajama bottoms
the Chicago Loop windows at Christmas
apple cider doughnuts
eerie lights
sitting down and really thinking about an
    attitude of yours that you are not sure
    is valid
taking a dare
feet sticking out of a sandpile
bare trees revealing each small movement
    of birds and animals
discussing philosophical matters of import
opening one's eyes a little more
fast learners
vast areas of cattails and river bulrushes
knowing what to do when the power fails
acorn squash
sauerbraten: pot roast marinated several
    days in vinegar with vegetables and
    spices
Zorro and the Lone Ranger

cherry vanilla flavor

judging a restaurant by its French fries

a rainbow of soap bubbles dancing across
the dishpan

changing self-defeating behavior

being soft-spoken

when your self-centered concerns shrink

"open studio" day

a misbuttoned shirt

Ben Affleck and Matt Damon

backgammon sets for four players

chili bowls with handles and lids

spice-colored kitchens

postcards from friends dear and far

night-lights in hotels

well-worn stone steps

list-lovers

center-cut bacon

curly endive

sunglasses with tortoiseshell frames

sitting on an outdoor patio overlooking a
duck pond

snow berries

fresh supplies of wood for the fire

amateur psychoanalysis

chowder of milk, potatoes, onion, salt
pork or bacon pieces

love: reaching, touching, caring, sharing
sunshine, showers and flowers; happy
hours together

archaeological sites
walls overgrown with a green cloak of ivy
congratulating a friend
variety being the spice of life
applying to graduate school
steamed clams, salad, and French bread
as a light summer dinner
asking advice from a youngster
good directions
sapphire mountains set into emerald
valleys
buffalo plaid
making yogurt
white clapboard houses
Special K cereal going great with fruit
slide rules
clear-glass candle cups
when people donate to support your
website
hubcaps
wearing three bracelets at a time
taking something off the grocery shelf,
deciding you don't want it, and then
putting it in another section
side dishes
searching out a piece of solitude and
refreshing yourself with the sound of
absolutely nothing
gearing up
being able to say, "I made it myself"

the creak and complaint of ice crystals
    shrinking upon themselves
velvety lemon mousse
the brake pedal on the passenger side of
    the car that you wish existed when
    you're riding with a lunatic
patchwork calico
treating yourself to orchestra seats for
    one performance
bread sliced slim as a leaf
a sense of continuity
people who take risks, who are creative
    and love to experiment, who improvise
    and make the best of what they have
Mamma Mia!
cork panels filled with art, ideas, fabric
    scraps, color swatches
coolers of cold cola
double-decker London buses
the quintessential lumberjack's breakfast,
    piled high, glistening with melted
    butter, dripping with maple syrup,
    and partnered with a few choice
    strips of bacon or plump sausages
Carl Sagan, astronomer
jumping-frog contests
the first blush of falling in love
an iron candle chandelier
a shampoo session outside
having a diamond re-set

toasting bagels

noise-canceling headphones

pounding surf

free refills on milkshakes

tastefulness

a weekend for two

Belgian endive and breadsticks for
scooping cheese

Oh, wow!

listing names and page numbers of
favorite recipes inside cookbook
covers

FAQs answered

pronouncing Oregon correctly

hotdogging stunts

sweet potatoes with a glaze of sugar,
cinnamon, margarine, and cornstarch

#1 or #2? A or B?

being surprised at what you learn about
yourself

purple crocuses with saffron-rich stamens

Mount Everest

the most inspiring place
you have ever been

very white tennis shoes and
very yellow tennis dresses

thick bark on the trees

tangerine juice

something wicked you find awkwardly
appealing

taking a "constitutional"
pinecones for kindling, bought at the
    roadside stand with pumpkins and
    Indian corn in the fall
working out at the gym
passion reciprocated
stars outside the airplane window
small steaks
Currier & Ives winter scenes
playing badminton
cold asparagus tarragon
"call waiting"
pastel skies
chickens in the dooryard
Kansas City barbecue style
discovering the philosopher's stone
Casablanca (movie)
baby formulas
a room under the eaves
being—or living with—an intuitive cook
Smokey the Bear
stockings hung on the shower rod
talking shop
the suitcase that keeps going around and
    around the baggage carousel
succotash: corn, beans, tomatoes, and
    cream
envelope purses
"No one else will ever love you the way
    I do."

your favorite hair product, hamburger
    accompaniments, high school
    memory, highway, holiday music,
    hot drink on a cold day, hotel,
    houseplant, hymn
something frothy as icing
dusk lingering with long light on the
    hilltops
families that spend leisure hours together
    having a chance to grow and
    understand one another
faucets and their handles
a bell to ring when you enter an office or
    a store
chunky tomato-dill soup
chase scenes
digging out an old family recipe
lemon and tropical spices
twirling a baton
fear of being approached by several dozen
    waiters singing "Happy Birthday"
leaving work early the day before a
    holiday
IBM's THINK motto
the Farrah Fawcett hairdo
roller-skating with a pillow strapped on
shaking up your routine way of doing
    things
an open bar
tasting menus

rolled-up shirtsleeves
when, for the moment, the
    crowd is somewhere else
playing house, school, restaurant as a kid
outdoor thermometers
giving away or selling things you never use
monks' robes
believing you can do anything
an intricate Fabergé egg, a world in a
    gilded walnut shell
glimpsing a yeti
"accidentally on purpose"
checking the dates of stuff in the
    refrigerator and cupboards
butter-fried ham and farmer cheese
    sandwiches
goose pimples
leaded-glass kitchen wall cabinets for
    displaying jars of home-canned jams
    and vegetables
a taproom with bare floors
library books
taking someone a bunch of violets
driving a forklift or backhoe
adytum, any secret place
the rusty greens of the hickories
having your hair braided
Internet memes
ragged rain clouds scudding over Long
    Island Sound

understatement
buttered sandwich buns
FaceTime and Google Hangouts
spareribs and egg rolls
playing favorite records and dancing
    wildly in the living room
Art Deco geometrics
food coloring in snow to make hair and
    eyes for snowmen
breakfast in a pale pink light
buying two Sunday papers
Irish fishermen's pullovers of heavy,
    cream-colored wool
pine needles tipped with teardrops of rain
genealogy charts
a door on a base, used as a coffee table
    or desk
joining a flying club
a baby plant
screened porches, unscreened porches,
    glassed porches, unglassed porches,
    with old wicker chairs, and pots
    of geraniums, bringing romance
    to summer
sponge diving
police officers and firefighters
Yale University
a funster
the rasp of a file
purchasing a painting that goes up in value

seeds changing to flowers

tunnel vision

picking the right stock to buy

impressive muscle definition

cafés along the blue water's edge

riding in a wheelbarrow

the height to which a cat's rear end can
    rise to meet the hand stroking it

ice-cream store posters

high-banked, one-car-wide lanes that
    lead to picture-postcard thatched
    villages

the fragrance of a summer rose

taking a bow

the system whereby one dog can quickly
    establish an entire neighborhood
    network of barking

apple peeling

slinky dresses

"tubby time"

dreaming of sinking into a comfortable
    chair

a bring-your-own-dish party

Johnson & Johnson's baby powder

someone to fix your computer problems

the particular way you fold your laundry

a unicorn with a golden horn and Borgana
    flower garland

being an usher at a wedding

refinancing at a lower interest rate

taking a blanket and something to ward
     off chills when you go to the dunes
mowing the lawn in your swimsuit and
     sneakers
open-mindedness
cereal-and-fruit parfaits
antique or old childhood books
rosemary-sage-myrtle herb candles in
     terra-cotta pots
Charlie Brown and Snoopy
the positive parts of your day
making lists at bedtime
a single flower floating in a small brandy
     snifter
loving freely, purely
apples and sweet potatoes with pork chops
knowing every minute counts
malted-milk waffles and pancakes
being delayed in an interesting airport like
     Dulles in Washington, D.C.
layer cakes
a friend who owns a truck
exploring your unconscious
enjoying a summer moon
children at recess
tree houses
Paul Revere's silver
Pizza Hut restaurants
puppet shows
a baby who sleeps through the night

blue jonquils

when an incumbent decides not to run
and the seat is fair game

getting out of debt

a rickety wharf, its legs stockinged in
barnacles

Dilbert (comic strip)

sack lunches

dining by the window

"Geronimo!"

cat food commercials

puttering about the house

recalling the smell of newly
mimeographed test papers

a contented elderly couple

par-3 golf

having something to read tucked in your
pocket or handbag

being partners

storm sashes

picking huckleberries on a hike

freezing bread dough

inheriting an island

oatmeal with maple crumbles on top

big, hooded trench coats

second chances

a college fund piggybank

candles glimmering behind cut-glass
holders that reflect the light
100 times over

hearing a sound you don't notice until it
    stops, like the furnace or refrigerator
to-go coffee and sandwiches
generosity
practicing 10,000 hours to learn
    something expertly
strange paw prints to investigate
a seafarer's knot
mouthwatering delicacies
Kentucky mints
squirrels with the bushiest tails
letting someone else shine
clean motels
a family of writers
Mountain Dew soda pop
summer glacier skiing in New Zealand
repairing a lamp
quarterbacks, even Monday-morning ones
knife-sharpened pencils
strawberry-flavored milk
true love
faith in yourself
Chanel quilted purses with chain straps
waking up in a hogan on an island in Canada
working "smarter"
having the number of a child's birthday
    party guests equal the child's age
a reassuring email
snow swirling on the road
marrying when the time is right

an empty parking space
candied sweet potatoes
good news
a field guide to happiness
the uses of a yardstick
a television set in an armoire
log cabin restaurants
sorting clean laundry
wrinkle-resistant clothes
heated sidewalks and driveways
study-hall escapades
bar napkins
beef cuts: pot roast, rib roast, brisket,
    chuck steak, club steak, Delmonico
    steak, Porterhouse, filet mignon, top
    sirloin, rib-eye, round steak, T-bone
baling hay
making plans
pie throwing
being happy together
flannel pants and long, crisp walks
beaches that are red in the east, honey
    in the middle, and tawny in the west,
    sloping gently to the water, backed
    by bluffs and dunes and cut by bays
    and harbors
every word in the lexicon
pan pizza from Domino's
a clock big enough to see without your
    glasses on

agreeing on the restaurant to go to and
the movie to see
railroad tracks
an attempt by a gumball to sneak out
of the chute and roll past the buyer
videos that you learn something from
chairs of bent bamboo and floors of cool
tiles
heartfelt apologies
Oriental rugs
the structure of texts
a ritual opening of the kilns each spring
The Palm Arbor Supply Company
the Grateful Dead, Pearl Jam, and Phish
having a tree house instead of a deck
going vegetarian a few days a week
liking the same foods as your partner
sunscreen for a boat ride
a kayak built for two
watermelon-rind pickles
the Qantas koala bear
the resonance of crystal
school pictures
the whoosh and roar of the wind
the silence of an electric car
daffodils and primroses rising from
the grass
wide pants
burnt-sugar chiffon cake
wild seascapes

controlling the largest empire on a
    Monopoly board
chartered buses for wrestling teams
doing something every year so that it
    becomes traditional
fresh, romantic, tender moments
being in a position to make a monetary
    donation
one remote control
apricot jelly-roll cake
atmospheric haze
cloth or paper kites
ground chuck
homemade penuche
Malcolm Gladwell's writing
quarts of milk
a sweet tooth
wading in the water after sleeping
    in the sun
remembering the wisdom you've been
    taught
leaning on a buck-and-rail fence
tiny sample perfume vials
laurel leaves
multicolored layered seeds and nuts
    in an apothecary jar
blind faith
the tangy scent of wax and varnish
bonus rooms
gathering around the piano in the lounge

a baseball card collection passed down to
    the next generation
picnic tables on the pier
taxi whistles
when a back or neck pain goes away
Jimmy Carter, former President
sand, soft underfoot
waking up with a really pleasant thought
burgundied meatballs and dilled
    mushrooms
the gleaming symmetry of a frosted
    spiderweb at dawn
bow-tie pasta
longtime couples who still enjoy each
    other's company
when the soup du jour at the corner deli
    is your absolute favorite
green-onion dip
iridescent shapes
sunlight making polka dots on noses as it
    spills down through oak leaves
smithing: arrow, black, blade, copper,
    gold, lock, pewter, silver, sword, tin
twin theaters
poor-boy shirts
being moved by a book or by nature
victory shouts
knowing you'll get seven hours of sleep
celebrating unusual holidays listed on
    your calendar

bebop tunes
early morning parkouring in the city
plaid cotton flannel
medical kits
keeping each thing to its season
chocolate milk
the rare movie that revisits your
    consciousness the next day
the four basic food groups
deep-sea fishing charters
writing to lots of people
army surplus
petrified wood
Winn-Dixie stores
sacks of spices
a hiatus
changing framed pictures for the season
dinners including choice of appetizer,
    salad, potato, and drink
winning an over/under bet
doing some research on the place you
    want to visit on your next vacation
shabby gentility
big data
your old Filofax agenda books
daisies exercising in the breeze
new potatoes baked in butter and sugar
escaping the grubby difficulties of real life
    into a more enticing fictional world
joining Habitat for Humanity

interesting cuff links

reserving a window table

eating a nutritious breakfast

naive art produced by someone untrained

really high voter turnout

violinists raising their bows

pulling a rocker close to the stove

Valentine's Day, the oldest holiday

ship models and nautical memorabilia

a well-executed U-turn

a content creator

the smell of bathroom soap

hors d'oeuvres small enough to eat in
one bite

a young forest in green pinstripes

a bubbling hot tub

spoon coasters

potted palms

bananas and orange juice

work that you love and that benefits
others

great escapes

a pen that writes when you start writing

playing fetch with a cat

big paychecks

fog: technically nothing but a cloud in
contact with the earth

having your gang meet for pictures at a
studio that takes turn-of-the-century
photos

a Qing Dynasty artist's brush jar
the Big Countdown on radio stations on
New Year's Eve
winter's ice-cream sea
using a sandglass instead of something
digital
sterling silver
playing Yahtzee
flatware with clear Lucite handles
yoga with a pet
Providence, Rhode Island
keeping the scorebook during a game
a sunken living room
stemmed bubble goblets
the most-consumed food products: milk,
cereal, bottled water, soft drinks,
bread, potatoes, beef, sugar
Highlights (children's magazine)
being all dressed up with somewhere to go
honeymooners wandering and exploring
their destination
closet offices
the serrated teeth of a tape dispenser
rakes, trowels, and spades
paddleboarding
inconspicuous consumption
Galileo slow thermometers: crystal orbs
rearranging themselves
a movie review that agrees with your view
the speed of light

going Botox-less

a rubber stamp printed with a favorite
slogan

pot roast gravy

kiss, kiss, hug, hug

64 new crayons

knowing the names of your senators and
representatives

a sled and team of horses for gathering
the sap, which is taken to the sugar
house for boiling down to syrup

drawing energy and vitality from one's
surroundings

a very old mulberry tree

miniature angel food cakes with frosting
in the middle

candles hooded with red parchment
shades

earthscape art, such as large geometric
drawings on beaches

never anticipating wealth from any source
but labor

slow curves

an eat-in-the-rough restaurant

chili in summer

annotation of lists

spending a night at a farmhouse

leisurely bubble baths

an ingenious ruse

free online lessons in almost every subject

when you walk right through a long
     roped-off lineup thing at an airport
     or a bank
a smilet
enduring traditions
the United States Geological Survey
     website and maps
chicken salad with apples, grapes, and
     celery
the green of white pines and firs and
     native spruces
soft-pile rugs
seventh-inning stretches
colorful fishing boats
cooking without an oven
planting a window box
Tightwad, Missouri
a peaceful chalet tucked away in nature
a potato salad recipe book
traveling through a bustling city
licorice sticks
knowing the best things in life are free
having a wonderful nurturing side
a Saturday morning round of clean-the-
     house
chairs with sidearm tables
rereading a good book
reed-fringed lagoons
fine cuisine
the simple life of worms

Velcroed toddler sneakers
the fairy-tale factory in your mind
the value of a hug from a loved one
getting married on February 29
the "armchair public"
the oboe
jump shots
takeout falafel
the texture of cream
sleeping on a train
cowlneck sweatshirts
thickets of blackberry bushes and
      morning glory vines
deviled ham and relish sandwiches
pundits/talking heads
the skillful articulation of a word's exact
      meaning
circle pins
executive jump ropes with digital counters
oil paintings
the high notes of an opera soprano
a dryer chuntering
Road Runner
an old family Bible
tortoiseshell headbands
thank-you notes
appliances in bright, surprising colors
a baptism
the *LOVE* sculpture by Robert Indiana
not cracking your knuckles

just happening upon a parking spot in the
    perfect place
box springs
putting on the sound track of a favorite
    Broadway show and singing in the
    shower or kitchen
wildcard teams
sleeping soundly when it's snowing hard
    at bedtime; waking full of anticipation
stoneware tortilla warmers
cracking a secret code
the tilde and the schwa
signing up for a makeover
a drumroll
beach lunches
rain forests
rocking chairs, more evocative than
    almost any other piece of furniture
locking glove compartments
granny nighties
an unexpected "yes"
bandeau tops
an isthmus (and the Little Rascals saying,
    "Isthmus be my lucky day!")
getting the best news of your life
the Greek alphabet: alpha, beta, gamma,
    delta, epsilon, zeta, eta, theta, iota,
    kappa, lambda, mu, nu, xi, omicron,
    pi, rho, sigma, tau, upsilon, phi, chi,
    psi, omega

rewarding yourself

walking a country lane on a cool morning

fruits that do not ripen after picking:
blackberry, blueberry, cherry, grape,
grapefruit, lemon, lime, litchi, orange,
pineapple, plum, raspberry, strawberry,
tangelo, tangerine, watermelon

the Farm Belt

a seven-point comfort check: brain,
temperature, light, noise, thirst,
digestion, body

a pulsating showerhead

blowing air out the window and seeing
steam

china cups and saucers

wind waltzing rain across the road

soundproofing

air hockey

slapping the bottom of a ketchup bottle
with the perfect intensity

self-acceptance

a friend with season tickets

the museum in your mind

free mints and toothpicks after dinner

tucking something special, like a little
note, into a lunch box, briefcase,
pocket, or purse

lying in bed at night, picking out one
thing you did well for the day, and
congratulating yourself

wearing one long braid

silky floss, antique lace

a kerfuffle

the first nip of clear, cold air

the sun bouncing off water

primping and powdering

getting to see what is in storage at an archaeological or natural history museum

pattern books for sewing clothes

a brainchild

crop rotation

watching a double feature at home

angel-food birthday cake

when the pink of the sunrise reflects on the snow of a glacier

3-D movies

herbs to use with cheese

the shape of a paint flake

the 2 percent of the Caribbean's numerous islands that are inhabited

warm-weather thirst quenchers

gift cards for a favorite restaurant

ice cream for dessert and coffee or lemonade

the Chiquita banana song

hunter-gatherers

potato fields

selling on consignment

golf links

unmowed patches of grass, discovered
  before one has put away the mower
Edwardian London
high-spired churches
teaching by example
remembering to write thank-you notes
standing at the window and seeing the
  snow, the flakes of crystal perfection,
  feathering from the sky
lemon pancakes served with fresh
  raspberries or raspberry syrup
summer theater
the way your lover looked at you the first
  time you met
historical buildings, quaint squares, and
  flower-trimmed alleys, all lined with
  restaurants and shops full of English
  woolens and china
instant-messaging services
pocket-size tissue packs
sucking it up
neon lights
the delicious cool of the uplands
soft, wet kisses and very big hugs
having a menu of reading with enough
  variety to ensure there is always
  something new to learn about
a small boy running into his mother's hug
breathing space
making toast with homemade bread

cobblestone streets

standing in the center of the Roman Colosseum

a barn busy with horses stamping and snorting

when the sky has lost the sunlight but not yet found the stars

Winter Carnival in St. Paul, Minnesota

vocabulary words known by heart

a volcano-shaped mound of mashed potatoes, gravy bubbling out from a deep crater formed by a heavy ice-cream scoop

unlikely juxtapositions

a heroic tale

equanimity

the word *boo*

the library's summer book club and earning gold stars

pajamas at breakfast

stately palms

the light inside the oven

your lifework

eating utensils

feeling gratitude in your bones

cutting alfalfa

brainstorming

toe clippers

exploring the twisting passageways of a limestone cave

Spandex
deep window ledges
blanket chests
browsing in a favorite book or electronics
    store
the patience to make pastries
spanakopita (spinach pie)
treating yourself to a new toothbrush
natural-wood milk pails
visualizing an impending occasion and
    considering all the pleasurable
    possibilities
brownie cake
sleeping in a back field
surfer havens
pulling a velvety petal from a flower and
    brushing it against your cheek
getting up first, making coffee, and
    delivering it to someone still in bed
old political cartoons
movie trailers
hybrid day, calla, and resurrection lilies
eight-foot-long scarves
pitting yourself against the wilds
your theory of the afterlife
the meaning of a bird's song
hamming it up
banjo pickers
when your street gets snowplowed
scrub pants

a checkers game set up atop a barrel
Portsmouth, New Hampshire
meeting the pilot
a squirrel's forepaws swiftly excavating a
    new hole
coral reefs, the marine equivalent of the
    rain forest
entertainers' real names
sight-reading music
driving up to the lake for a weekend with
    your pals
cosmic time
watching the sun fill the sky with colors
a sample flight of microbrewery beers
teas tailor-made to individual requirements
cleaning out the medicine cabinet
dancing dragons with up to 50 martial arts
    dancers inside
fresh paint
prepping your bath with scented sachet
    cubes, bubble bath, soaps shaped like
    shells
the Nobel Peace Prize winners
halter tops
mugs as pencil holders
Northern Exposure (TV show)
painting the town red
in cold weather, simmering apple cider,
    cinnamon, cloves, and tangerines to
    make the house smell cozy

early evening birdcalls

turning a plush bath sheet into a sarong

Lucite clipboards

a rainbow seen as a complete circle

professionally ironed hair

music without lyrics

bare trees spreading mantillas of black
    lace against the pale sky

mushroom identification

uncirculated pennies

a swimming pool at the hotel

tides breathing messages of change

Superman's red cape and blue tights

avocado plants

observing the guts of the creative process

baking potatoes in aluminum foil

serving warm, soft pretzels to guests who
    come expecting ordinary snacks

chenille sleeping socks with nonskid
    bottoms

collecting milk bottles

birds finding food in the winter

a walking stick

the sandpaper-like nubs on a cat's tongue

homemade stuffed mushrooms

NASA astronauts learning volcanic
    geology while preparing for lunar
    landings

"Ninety-nine may say no, the hundredth,
    yes."

sitting on a stoop, watching dusk change
        to darkness and counting the stars
golf books
double-bolting the door
layered salad
the dew, the air, the sounds of the birds
the half-lotus position
baby corncobs
keyboard shortcuts
a carefully arranged mind
flaming-bright maple trees
receiving a promotion
glazing a pot
fashion quizzes
dawn chorus
length, width, depth, and time
ditto marks
the collar never folded down on a cotton
        turtleneck
"egg in snow" with smoked bacon
cubic zirconia
being cautious
school mascots
markers from Civil War battlefields
a blend of toothpaste and mouthwash
cos (romaine) lettuce
sipping a Coke
fasting on warm milk and sweet
        bread the night before turkey
yummy-to-lick envelopes

blueberries and raspberries to freeze for
winter pies

lava lamps' guck blobs

"Free Bird" (Lynyrd Skynyrd)

your grandparents' Florida room

museums devoted to unusual topics

the smell of vinegar and pickling spices
drifting out the door

the abyssal zone

quarter-zip sweaters

lakeside roads with farm stands offering
apples, pumpkins, pears, and other
fruits and vegetables

achieving more, but possibly doing less,
with rest

the last glow of the fireplace

small tidal pools in which you can see
bright green moss and species of
marine life

Gustave Stickley, Duncan Phyfe, and
other famous cabinetmakers

circular couches

apricots to zucchini

colorful, one-cushion loveseats

blowing out all the candles

balancing the checkbook at a sidewalk
café

serpentine-link necklaces

a word you always mistype, like
"something" or "cushion"

cyclists who wear their helmets

kindly given instruction

taking the time to be appreciative

unhurried hours away from pressures

nurturing creativity

bold, exciting looks

passing a test

a sandstone landscape being set alight by
the setting sun

beach babies

world-class photographers

koi pond fish

longhorn cheese

"It will rain if cows are lying down in the
pasture."

two-for-one sales

notched-collar blazers

taking back-road tours

a beautiful old hotel in London

wind heard at the chimney and around the
corners of the house, swishing and
roaring through the naked woodland
and sighing among the pines and
hemlocks

extravagant lawn parties

at a 6 a.m. breakfast, watching the sky
perform

using a table of contents or a short,
out-of-context chapter to spark
a new kind of logic

graceful sofas with slightly faded covers
setting aside time for relaxation
stone fireplaces
bright, sunny cold days
cypress trees
a bulletin-board collage
freebies and cheapies
premoistened towelettes
block parties
being amused by the antics of one's pets
ground beef
the thumping sound of a wheelbarrow
Twitter tweets
the pentathlon
the sweet victory of all the gears in your
      brain turning at the right time in the
      right place
"Nice socks!"
muffins coming cleanly out of paper
      holders
small-town cafés
the small bar that turns an "O" into a "Q"
hoarding the licorice jellybeans
letter sweaters and pleated skirts
passion flowers
not-overpowering scented candles
the fogging of bathroom mirrors
wearing your best color
the smell of onions and sausages cooking
baby cougars

anything and everything well-made
the five Great Blessings: Happiness,
    Health, Virtue, Peace, Longevity
a wonderful restaurant that few people
    know about
bucking a trend
being prankish
police car loudspeakers
preventive medicine
seaside communities
special art exhibits
the first paragraph of a newspaper article
looking up obscure words others use in
    Scrabble
curds and whey
living life spontaneously
First Night
panini sandwiches and wine flights
rain rivers
when the hot dogs come in an eight-pack
    and the buns in a six-pack
your own llama
doing something posthaste
the complex, the nuanced, the sloppy
antitrust laws
vacuum bottles
steel-belted radial tires
your favorite earrings, egg dish, Elvis
    song, encyclopedia, ethnic food,
    exercise, expensive date

litmus paper
double rainbows
Halley's Comet
handwoven fabrics, tinted with rich,
    earthy colors from the juices
    of fresh berries
kirigami and origami
sweater coats
looking at old family photos
burnishing your own philosophy
a waving tide of color
diagramming a sentence
the one cube left by the person
    too lazy to refill the ice tray
crazy hats and sunglasses
white ash tennis rackets
guided imagery
double shoelace knots that you can untie
    easily
the invention of contact lenses
the swirly, splotched-paint pictures you
    can make at a fair
laughing at someone's attempt at
    watermelon growing
insalata verde
pinecones dropping in the fall
Breathe Right nose strips
an auctioneer's hammer
South Dakota: Badlands, Black Hills,
    Mt. Rushmore, clear days

duck decoys
the pasteurization process
preserving rain forests
wet babies
a great date movie
Aesop's Fables
white porcelain cups and saucers
    sprinkled with delicate confetti dots
anticipation being the greater joy
striking while the iron is hot
a fleet of taxis when you need one
an ice-cream table and chairs
someone to kiss goodnight
little paper cups of honey butter
tactful lighting, like apricot-pink
golfing with fathers
raking leaves
$1 Washington, $2 Jefferson, $5 Lincoln,
    $10 Hamilton, $20 Jackson, $50 Grant,
    $100 Franklin, $500 McKinley,
    $1,000 Cleveland, $5,000 Madison,
    $10,000 Chase, $100,000 Wilson
selling your first house
making cut flowers last
oversized bathtubs
a butter crock
morning light
room at the inn
airy eggnog
ice buckets

an occasional trash breakfast, like a bowl
    of Trix and a dip into a juicy novel
hula, lei, muumuu, ukulele, luau
the foxtrot
skinless all-beef kosher hot dogs
a treasure hunt for red raspberries or
    running vine blackberries
candlelight ceremonies
the whack of a bat against a baseball
guitar lessons
fascinating facts
an atomic alarm clock
music that comforts you
the zip-p-p of a zipper
Monopoly games
corn and potato chowder
beginning a journal in a blank book
an unbusy mall
honesty being the only policy
"There's an app for that . . ."
Weekly Reader (magazine)
a lynx on a Rocky Mountain crag
shirttails hangin' out
the ways people stand at a corner
riding a bobsled course
rub-on, wash-off tattoos
responsible babysitting
a cat stropping its claws on the post you
    provided
Yankee ingenuity

the shaded quiet of a Victorian gazebo and
the tranquility of the woods
etiquette observation
a three-year-old's imagination
acts of kindness, no matter how small,
never being wasted
Chase's Calendar of Events (book)
cultivating the habit of success
listening to your silent voice
large, messy submarine sandwiches
avenues of majestic trees
being grateful
country fairs
extra-virgin olive oil
emerald islands
remembering your sunglasses
soccer socks
supper dances
Toygers and perma-kittens
angst subsided
Labor Day weekend
successfully defending your thesis
saddle-soaping leather
"once in a blue moon"
catching a robber
being ready for your close-up
apple wedgers and corers
crumpets, straight-sided, pale, round and
hot, honeycombed with holes ideal
for absorbing butter

popcorn stitching
interpreters and period singers
miter boxes
finding a 4,600-year-old city in Peru
a turkey sauce of cooked cranberries and
     ground whole oranges
candlelight dinners at eight instead of
     neon-lit dinners at six
pistachio muffins served warm
John Lennon and Paul McCartney,
     musicians
birdies singing the same song over and over
society girls
playing Password
prosciutto and melon
setting a watch or clock fast in an
     effort to be more punctual
thick sweaters
cotton candy
congratulatory notes
homecoming festivities
Bert and Ernie (from *Sesame Street*)
doodads
dill weed from California
the humanities
greenhouse-fresh roses
a red brick factory with a waterwheel
walking barefoot in the park
a reflective turn of mind and a special spirit
     of enjoyment found in New England

cave-dark pubs

rating movies and books online so you get
    appropriate recommendations

overstuffed sandwiches

camel caravans

Tarzan, Texas

Christmas crackers

touring the Galápagos and reading Darwin
    on the spot

breaking even

a toy that moos when you turn it over

dinner bells

playing games in a cool basement during
    summer

free community resources—libraries,
    talks, etc.

ornament storage boxes

a lit-from-within glow

drive-in movies

beauty lessons

buying all new spices

that object you wouldn't trade for the world

the first frost coming without a whisper,
    the glistening leaf, the gleaming vine

old-fashioned washboards

a June-in-February party

bread-and-butter pickles in blue-tinted
    Mason jars

men who explain their behavior by saying,
    "I'm just a wild 'n' crazy guy!"

Bozo the Clown
getting caught singing to Muzak
     when taken off hold
everything
a cathedral of trees
helping conduct a census
paths edged with hibiscus
popping cheese cubes
the room tone or wildtrack, the barely
     audible noises that make up a
     background sense of quiet
hoisting the sails in Florida on brisk blue
     early mornings at the marina
first steps
taking care of plants
imagining a fire hydrant is a Martian in
     disguise
setting things in motion
the do-something-you-haven't-done-in-
     years plan
eating potato skins for the vitamins
an osprey nesting site
squirrels with question-mark tails, burying
     nuts in the lawn
ancient cities that people still live in
fortune cookies
miniature teacups and saucers
pea jackets
a mentor gently steering you in the right
     direction

glass apothecary jars with multicolored or
    different-shaped shells
pre-steaming fresh young vegetables—
    zucchini, yellow squash, corn on the
    cob, mushrooms—and then grilling
    them for a woodsy smoke flavor
things you can do with your eyes closed
a bush's shadow on a tree trunk
contributing to a lending library
corn-on-the-cob dishes
obi sashes
country mist
exchanging restaurant recommendations
    at breakfast
an old movie on a cold night
daffodils popping up in February and
    roses that bloom all year
turned-up shirt collars
Air Force One
the annual crane migration
standing up for yourself
noise, discord, and jargon reverberating
    and then settling like dust
the perfectly soft inside of a new
    sweatshirt
dairy cows
Debussy's *Clair de lune*
jeans with clean patches
a brand-new mattress
choral singing

timing your garage sale perfectly

Radio City Music Hall

dayspring, first light

being in the pink

putting your feet up

squooshing ice-cream sandwiches

being a benefactor

piggybacking errands

lemon Cokes

setting the scene, arranging the props,
and inviting your wittiest, chattiest
acquaintances

pretest jitters

braising food

really thick eyelashes

mullein, wild yarrow, broom sedge, and
dock

stationery embossers

French-milled soap, fresh flowers, and fruit

View-Masters and their reels

artists' pencils

pocket fishing poles

an introductory offer

colored bottles

window seats and bready-smelling mazes
of book racks

school songs

pooping out completely

kitchens with high ceilings and louvered
windows

daddies cooking dinner
baking-powder biscuits
the difference between algae and fungi
storyboarding a comic strip
years from now, remembering everything:
    the light, the words said, the magic
    mood
a comfort station
perfect baked potatoes
goo-goo eyes
getting up and watching the sun rise
    even if you don't have to because
    of your job
treating everyone with civility and respect
complimentary appetizers of barbecued
    meatballs and cheese spread served
    with melba toast
photographing the changes of season
no line at the returns desk
fresh, free, and sensitive people
unused paints
Brie en brioche
flight bags
newspaper stylebooks
spinning pennies
the area on a windshield that the wipers
    can reach
Wrigley's gum
moon tides
sand cats of the Sahara Desert

natural pine paneling and shutters
ESPN SportsCenter
secret closets
fuzzy rugs
apricot sunsets
affordable hair extensions
playing patty-cake
twenty magazines for your vacation
light, silver-dollar-size sour-cream
    hotcakes
businessmen's striped Oxford shirts
bridal showers
pleasant autumn drives
the momentary confusion experienced
    when you hear a cell phone ringing
    and wonder whether it is yours
a price sticker that peels off completely
jogging with a friend
giving others ample opportunity to speak
treadle sewing machines
six-lane freeways
the first crossword puzzle, 1913
red velvet cake
staying until the candle burns out
inviting a new acquaintance to breakfast
a sharp paring knife
columnists who run out of ideas
waitress uniform dresses
raffia sun hats
the day slipping away

reversing a hair permanent

toy planes made of balsa wood

homemade soup: bubbling softly, warming
the house with delicious aromas, and
comforting your tummy on chilly
nights

riding around town on roller skates

working in an electronic cottage

office file cabinets

cuddly white rabbits

wrapping gifts

smoking-hot biscuits

a breakthrough

Totes umbrellas and overshoes

wallpaper decorated with roses

raspberries picked in the garden

an estimated 16.5 million people
celebrating their birthday each day

speaking loudly to foreigners as if
somehow it makes you easier to
understand

lemon shake-up drinks at the fair

wagon-wheel chandeliers

swamp maples in bright red, yellow,
orange, and crimson flames

wabi-sabi: imperfect, impermanent,
incomplete objects

"Let's see what we find in the fridge."

chopped wood ready to go

little boys' spiraled curls ruffling up

when you're in love with the world
times when you have to eat and run
using a razor
the helpful illustrations in cookbooks
a weekend gathering spot
bowls of sparkling berries and fresh
      cream, baskets of popovers and
      croissants with little pots of jams and
      jellies, steaming coffee and freshly
      squeezed orange juice, thick country
      bacon, hot maple syrup, pancakes,
      and French toast
setting sail
drawing hopscotch lines
music in the air
your firstborn
the plethora of computer languages
phone calls from far away
sheepish smiles
a fun-to-be-fit attitude
melt-away mints
whatever you're good at
triple sheets and show pillows
silver whistles
a pond so placid it mirrors a willow tree
sling pumps
dress-down days
Herculean feats
the ability to persist
neural networks

forty winks
nuclear disarmament
using the drive-through window
logs and fires
bright green peas and broccoli in a
    Chinese restaurant
a traditional cross-country sled
researching a business venture
a single bird making a graceful descent
    and perfectly timed splashdown
giving a briefcase to someone who really
    needs one
furry booties that warm your feet like
    little ovens
fixing gourmet meals
a decathlon champion
quiet green courtyards
a bench at the foot of the bed that rolls on
    casters for dining and writing
memories that revolve around food
alpacas, humming sheep
fluorescent-lit luncheonettes
a barbecue sauce poised between
    molasses sweetness and spicy tang
happy socks
double locks
chess sets that invite competition
stuffed pizza, descendant of Chicago's
    famous deep-dish pizza
microfiber cleaning cloths

a perfectly harmonized national anthem
shiny hair
the Magi's gold, frankincense, and myrrh
Tod's and Gucci handbags
the nickname "Bear"
country stores
walking shady paths in the woods
     surrounding the inn
decorating with sheets
having the ducks at the zoo eat the bread
     you've thrown to them
providing incentives and rewards
lab smocks
baseball terms
Bunker Hill
a catamaran cruise to a private beach
painting pictures of your garden flowers
trying on something that is too big
fresh air and good food
New York: Manhattan, Catskills, Niagara
     Falls, Statue of Liberty, upstate
the sugar-scented green of leaves
throwing your hair back away from your
     face to feel the sun
rotisseries: Ferris wheels for chickens
sleepy babies and teddy bears
casino parties
learning astronomy
poets using words to convey what lies
     beyond words

the things we don't talk about for fear that
    people won't understand
ignoring unconstructive criticism
garden ferns
brewing a pot of cinnamon coffee
vegetarian restaurants
the tolling of a church bell
hoping to have another bestselling book
"Barbara Ann" by the Beach Boys
marital fidelity
a sunny place set up for lunch
Edith Piaf records and café au lait
wind-combed goldenrod
homemade soap bubbling in an iron pot
    on the hearth
an old farm table in the kitchen
silver trays of fresh fruit grouped in fans
    and slices
Maryland: National Anthem, Annapolis,
    crabs, horses, Camden Yards
exercising immediately after work
misting indoor plants
Santa Claus
massive grain bins awaiting the harvest
    from fields of high corn
the mountaintops of love
Daisy Hill Puppy Farm, where Snoopy
    was born
a comeback for culottes
writing your name in fresh cement

naked maples casting black shadows

water hyacinths

packing a two-week wardrobe in a carry-
on bag

the Rubik's Cube and the Magic 8-Ball

a Cape Codder

holiday petits fours

Yosemite National Park

modular storage systems

arranging a work area

dormitory life

beach scenes

stair treads

a pond right in front of a home

the way every reader discovers in the
same words a different story

the button at the top of a baseball cap

getting writing advice from someone
whose writing you love

glass-bottomed boat rides

shell blouses

Frito pie: chili, cheese, corn chips; maybe
salsa, sour cream, rice, jalapeños

fresh lemonade made from squeezed
lemons, water, and sugar

the human ear maintaining our sense
of balance (equilibrium) and
coordination of head and eye
movements

top-opening notebooks

the plethora of images on the Internet
intaglio printing
the one leaf still clinging to the tree on
    January 1
a solid-pine drop-leaf table
Blondie and Dagwood
a woman wearing a men's size 10½ shoe
a farewell episode of a TV show
the spirit of childlike eagerness
rib-eye steaks for lunch
a quiet area in an office building
the waves on top of a meringue pie
mulling spices of stick cinnamon, dried
    sweet orange peel, cracked nutmegs,
    and whole cloves
Brazilian coffee
homemade Easter eggs
a polar ice cap
the National Guard
celebrating self-invented holidays
being someone's knight in shining armor
jack-in-the-box music
jungle gyms
crocheted snowflakes
garden gnomes
seagulls sailing over the dunes
Noah's Ark
books full of years of research
learning the language
valuable stock options

chain stores
travel or disposable toothbrushes
sparkling French blue and soft peach
    Spanish poppies
a favorite pen
when you finally see the car that's coming
    to pick you up
renting a bike
dinner service
the valedictorian and salutatorian
tubes of paint in wooden crates
washing your hair
when the tollbooths are removed
those revered for mischief
Paleolithic rock art sites
a multigeneration cookbook
sweethearts
the remote control in your possession
a feline exploring new territory
rabbit tracks in the snow
diamond rings
learning everything you possibly can
    about a subject that interests you
a snap in the air in fall
third markdowns
guarding your private time as your most
    treasured asset
northern New England's mud season
pumpkins heaped at the roadside stand
spring skiing

pillow fights, blanket tents, spooky
    stories, dressing up the cat
a glass hors d'oeuvre server with sections
    for dips
pullout trays and foldout pantries
impatiently popping toast up and down in
    the toaster
high-shuttered windows
studying, capturing, cataloging the things
    that make life rich
a force of nature
bangs for a high forehead
castle-hopping
knowing why
plaid skirts
shatter-resistant Plexiglas
the sound of a priest chanting
tools impacting civilization: knife, abacus,
    compass, pencil, harness, scythe,
    rifle, sword, eyeglasses, saw, watch,
    lathe, needle, candle, scale, pot,
    telescope, level, fish hook, chisel
enormous striped lollipops from highway
    rest areas
fewer diet books on the bestseller list
confetti-tossed hair
cat toy makers in Vermont
soft-sided luggage
weaving black-ash baskets
double-decker sandwiches

bright rubies
new life
a short but sweet summer
comedy records
the cool underside of a pillow
being centered
growing one's nails for special occasions
(like receiving a ring)
Continental breakfasts
the flat wooden "spoons" that come with
ice-cream cups
a wall of books
stopping to rest under the drooping shade
of a river's edge willow tree
waiting for the team bus
middle age
cruising on a skateboard
the act of worship
seeing eye to eye
homemade English muffins
oatmeal raisin cookies
old-fashioned waffle-weave kitchen towels
treasure hunts
a baby falling asleep
the TV Guide channel
a menu of "little bites" and "big bites"
butterscotch-striped swimsuits
Christmas trees lining the street, their
lights reflecting in the frost that
covers the cobblestones

knowing "it's always something"

butter on every bite

watching football practice

gatehouses converted into beautiful, grand
entrances to manor houses or estates

with camera and binoculars in hand,
putting your feet up on the rail and
settling back to watch the harbor
drama unfold

thermal blankets

moving to a better place

a tribe of goldfish flicking their tails

a popular girl

kisses: love's punctuation marks

juniper berries

punctuality

a boss who lets you be autonomous

potato patties filled with meat and onion

billiard and pool parlors

the playground of life

all 1,440 minutes in a day

an après-ski atmosphere

enjoying a glass of iced tea under the
grape arbor

getting a puppy

Canadian pro football

snowflakes twirling through the treetops

particle physics

a bathroom with mirrored walls, scented
soaps, and great fluffy towels

eyes entranced by the play of sunlight on
the water
coffee, tea, or milk
an olive stoner
personalized compacts
your definition of "wild"
eating after brushing your teeth
an old covered bridge
sleigh bells
fresh pea soup in a restaurant
Romance, West Virginia
nautical knots
the fullest day of summer
living in a tree house
getting a family heirloom fixed
helping someone less fortunate
pleated lampshades
Vivaldi in the morning
knowing the Heimlich maneuver and CPR,
even though you never want to use
them
those with business acumen
opening a paintbox of brilliantly colored
chunks
an encampment of tepees, lean-tos, and
pioneer wagons
open-hearth baked ham
the tart-sweet, sharp-clean scent of
lemons and oranges in the air
a movie studio lot

a string of really bad luck finally being
    broken
celebrating the harvest moon by taking a
    long stroll with someone special after
    dinner or heading to the beach with
    warm blankets and wine
the be-all and end-all
opening lines of books
cleaning windows with squeegees
night football games
a bevy of eclectic sights
a map that's easy to follow
leaf-pickup days
a healed blister
being on time to classes
local color
squishy bags of pizza dough
crickets at dusk
laughing till you cry
travel mugs
snipping sun-bleached peppergrass next
    to the river
creamed carrots
hairy traffic dissipated
forming hands into a steeple
having small picture books, magazines,
    quick reads for guests
limbering up for sports
no-bean chili
cool, cooler, coolest

getting excited when talking about your
     work
trees: the quick-change artists of fall
Tennis, Kansas
knowing there will be many surprises in
     the future
music stands
antelope roaming
umbrellaed tables set out on a sunny pier
visiting someone you haven't seen in a
     very long time
brown bread
motionlessness
black bean and corn dip
risotto with butter and Parmesan
a farmers' market tailored to the kind of
     cooking you do
being told you're dazzling
barefoot beach barbecues
packets of tissues
the warbling of a canary
daytime dramas
"Nothing Books," blank books
     for writing
putting greens
a serenading minstrel
folding combs
mutual agreement
sketching trees in the backyard or in
     nearby woods

getting time from a parking meter that
   still has someone else's money in it
phases of growth
the ninth inning
bowling lawns
all the nuances of human character
ancient Egyptian mummies
munching cookies and sipping milk
coat styles: blanket, Chesterfield, duffel,
   pea, princess, swing, toggle, trench,
   wrap
post-prom breakfast and a walk on the
   beach
Sunday brunch buffet
getting to know people
Holland bulbs
hanging socks on your body because they
   have static electricity
food coloring mixed with egg yolk for
   painting food
a fun person with a good appetite,
   interesting work, good storytelling
   ability, slightly twisted humor, fresh
   insight, brave choices
staying in the tub longer than it takes to
   get clean
frost flowers
automobile airbags
admitting you were wrong
breath clouds on cold morning walks

effects of the smell of musk

a hanging place for wursts, bagged
cheeses, and strings of peppers

a minaudière

ravishing beauty

wearing pajama pants to work from home

the Basketball Hall of Fame in
Springfield, Massachusetts

picnic brunch

dreamy music

long hands

secret diaries

street lamps festooned
with garlands and bright bows

the South Pacific of James Cook

the high voice one uses when summoning
a cat

the first pleasant thoughts that go through
your mind the moment you awake

any lucky find, like money in a pocket

getting rid of a headache

gentlemen rising when a lady enters or
leaves a room

bamboo plates

a cardinal's brilliance against the snow

new cutlery

air-conditioning

a bouquet of straw flowers in a big basin
aglow with bee lights

your kinfolk

a penny on the pavement
the phony decor in an aquarium that
    fools fish into thinking they're in an
    underwater paradise
screwball comedy
advertisements with beautiful pictures
    of food, water droplets, something
    caught in motion
nursery school
recognizable noises at night
cats making velvet semicircles of
    contentment on the pillows
Connecticut: saltboxes, church spires,
    village greens, postcard towns
snow days when you're a child
French Canadian pea soup
semper fi
keeping the lights dim
hot, hot water
chicken or turkey salad sandwiches
making love after a party
holiday window gels
the Emmys
Muenster cheese
beach gear
mental alertness
needle-nose pliers
a rainbow of relishes
the cry of a killdeer
brown sugar melting over fresh pineapple

que pasa?
requesting the pleasure of a dance
access roads
El Dorado
the creative power of everything that exists
a bed that doesn't squeak
LED lights
feeling shy and wild
earthquakes that are exciting but don't
    do damage
babies' quilts
something new and bright to wear
full moons and black cats
wall-hung plate racks, a true country
    custom
finishing what you start
quiet neighbors
regular hedges of fruit trees, covered
    with beautiful flowers early in spring,
    charged with noble fruits in summer
    and autumn
back-saver snow shovels
a sense of dignity
yellow cheeses, fresh brown eggs, glowing
    pumpkins, tangy russet apples, farm
    butter proudly stamped with the
    maker's own mark, fat purple turnip
    globes, superb smoked hams, chicken
    with the flavor of Sunday afternoon
    family dinner, from local markets

a home chock-full of crafts and
   conversation pieces
luminous skin
researching and planning getaway
   weekends
wailing along with Aretha Franklin
venture capital
someone who says you're beautiful
winning a most-improved award
the aroma of cinnamon or bread that lures
   you to countless bakeries
entering your name in a local sweepstakes
indicating with a long-pronged fork that
   one of the steaks on the grill is "yours"
white cupcakes with multicolored sprinkles
walking tall
jumping rope to a skip-rope jingle
roast beef sandwiches with lettuce,
   mayonnaise, salt and pepper
a food you never eat except in restaurants
playing hooky to do something you don't
   ordinarily have time for
a fulcrum and lever
a smile on your driver's license photo
the elegance of white gloves
summer vegetable gardens
college basketball teams
Dutch apple pie, made of the thinnest
   apple slivers with a topping of butter
   crumbs

a set of premises
snow accumulating on the grass
picking out landmarks
little scoops of shade in sandy footprints
layers of sweatering
match point
getting a tan on the fire escape
arranging a platter of fruit or cheese
singing voices: alto, baritone, baritenor,
bass, basso profundo coloratura,
contralto, dramatic soprano, lyric
soprano, male soprano, mezzo-
soprano, soprano, and tenor
raised potato biscuits
having nine lives
carousels with music
a quiet day with the kids
scarlet flowers in hair
the desperation of a love letter
direct sunlight
honeymoons
when you drop a glass and it doesn't
break
meat carved into beautiful slices and
the fluffy mashed potatoes awaiting
abundant, flavorsome gravy
successful soul-searching
feeling like a child who thinks he's
mastered the art of shoe-tying
antique books

summer languor giving way to a sense of
purpose
Freeport, Brunswick, and Camden, Maine
Pierre Le-Tan's artwork
the crackle of new money
dance skirts
dreaming of going home
living in a lighthouse
wild ululation
Vancouver, British Columbia
kids with their T-shirts on backward,
sleepy over toast and jelly
good karma
a watercolor of the Maine landscape:
rocky terrain and sparse foliage, lit by
a full moon
treasure boxes
reading while taking a bath
a boy who follows in his mother's
footsteps
parachutes in the air
windows looking out on acres of
woodland
clever or cheerful mug mottos
an idyllic quiet broken only by the ripple
of the stirring water, the splash of
fish rising to flying insects, and the
crackle of a driftwood campfire
classic baklava
feeding a cat

glassed-in cupboards

lemon butter

the overwhelming desire to pop
someone's bubble-gum bubble

knotcraft and ropecraft

endlessly winding backroads

a new lens for your 35mm camera

getting into a bed with clean sheets right
after shaving your legs

a phenomenon like "Life is good"

"singing" greeting cards by Hoops and Yoyo

splurging on fresh flowers, flowering
plants, scented candles, and a fresh
batch of magazines

the promise of a small package

chilled soup in the summer

an in-flight phone call

a "dream team"

masked balls

things as plain as day

shin-kicking fun

sun reflecting the cove waters

Chocolat (the movie and the sound track)

corner-fitting desks or TV stands

the hearty shout of labor

gentle, rocking motion

votive candles

tomato paste in a tube

personal investigation and
experimentation

a credenza
do-it-yourself projects
a segue in language, like from TV dinners
    to frozen dinners
mobile homes
taking a flashlight wherever you go
jumping over the widest puddle
the funny feeling that you already put
    sugar in your coffee
a princess crown
your nest egg
peg-leg jeans, penny loafers, bobby socks,
    sloppy joe sweaters
cast parties
spaciousness
meat loaf seasoned with oregano, basil,
    minced onion, and nutmeg
Duraflame logs for the fireplace
an opulent third-century town house with
    a colonnaded courtyard
Whynot, Mississippi
once-in-a-lifetime chances
an honest answer
gift shops
watching as a raging ocean rises
reframing your thinking
unspoiled forests of oak, pine, magnolia,
    and palmetto
the excitement of viewing a meteor
    shower

the alternating pink and yellow sponge
   squares of Battenberg cake
baskets balanced on heads
a splurge
a graduation quilt made out of a kid's
   old T-shirts
alma maters
balcony- and shutter-trimmed houses
handling money
sharing a book you enjoyed
crisp fritters dipped in warm maple syrup
food prepared at hibachi tables
heather-cloaked heights
going to the country armed with books
   and a vision of autumnal walks and
   sunlit garden swings
the longer hairs of the pelt
lunch-counter cooking
figuring out port and starboard
lofty elms
wonderfully simple things
the three-way lightbulbs you save because
   at least one wattage still works
a baby in a floppy white hat
onion dicers
a confetti of light falling through leaves
charitableness
a blastoff
an incorrigible browser of goods
self-instruction

antique woodworking tools

a grand pooh-bah

wrapped-bodice, cowl-neck, or raglan-sleeve leotards

the right place at the right time

undulating cane fields

any party with a piñata

painted wood carousel lions from the late 19th century

macaroni jars

Bambi's rabbit friends

apricot shortbread pie with a glass of milk

sewing circles

newspaper delivery

the stop you make 15 feet from the pickup window to make sure your takeout order is all there and to put your money away

the weeds going berserk and lawns growing way too fast

pinch bowls

science books for laypeople

falling asleep on the lawn chair

the solid sound of a good car door shutting

the origin of the saying "no worries" (Australia, 1965)

emailing a photo to a faraway friend

the infinite possibilities of a sandwich

your amigos

the cardboard rod on a hanger that
   prevents creasing in pants
appliance carts when you need them
flea-market furniture
a more-than-happy feeling
people who ask you trivia questions
   instead of trying to make conversation
a day trip to an uncrowded place
a bowl of cornflakes and cold milk
spotting poison ivy's three leaflets
shelves lined with ancient tins and boxes
   holding their original contents
grouping chairs around a fireplace or near
   windows
soft, summery ivory light
a salad with an interesting house dressing
the munching of golden ears of corn
swimming in a natural brook across the
   road from an inn
hand-wrapped silk flowers in a willow
   basket
running a corporation
going to a local college football game with
   friends, even if no one attended the
   college
the quiet hush of a forest
taking a covered-wagon vacation in Kansas
artificial turf
the opposite of a backlog: work
   completed before it is required

a state of temporary quiescence
the only sounds at night being the
    conversations of tree frogs, crickets,
    and owls
a handful of raisins
bulldog tenacity
tiny condiment containers with room-
    service food
being one number away from bingo
Mr. Magoo, Charlie, and McBarker
luggage racks
Earth Day
not being too grown up for anything
ears of rabbits
photocopier enlargers
chrome on bikes
artesian wells
kidskin and snakeskin
ski mittens
cloud-watching
having the Sunday funnies on hand
pizza parlors
the science of sound
the smell of the sea
tulips, then apples, then peonies blooming
a Victorian bay window, a big four-poster
    bed with a blue-and-white quilt
rooftop heliports
who, what, where, when, why, and how
driving through a giant sequoia

displaying paintings on easels
sitting beside a fire and hearing wind tides
    suck at the chimney, swish against
    the corner of the house, and quiver
    the panes
meaningful and telling winks
runcible spoons
braised sirloin of beef Beaujolais
full freezers
cane and bamboo
the fragrant worlds of Crabtree & Evelyn
    and Caswell-Massey
an outboard motor gargling at dawn
bike baskets
poetry's nonutilitarian nature
your brain's dictionary
underwater limestone formations
eating meals
whole carrots baked in honey
a special weekend event
mint sprigs
the atmosphere of family chain
    restaurants
drifting on a raft
inexpensive formal gowns
the glow you get from being outdoors
heavy diner mugs
pitchers on the porch
clear blue bays
soft, buttery things

driving an old pickup truck

shimmering blue lakes

a set of sharpened colored pencils on
your desk in a glass for doodling and
jotting notes in something other than
gray lead

the light between the slats of the blinds

eating an exotic fruit or untried vegetable

elk bugling in the cool autumn air

zippy limes

playing a sport whole-hog

bike-decorating contests

spray-on deodorant

a short, squat candle in a tart tin

sliding back and forth in the bathtub in
order to mix the too-hot water with
the cooler water

meeting eyes

combining mustards

thumb indexes

challah bread

juice served in champagne flutes

double agents

homemade stationery

to go for a rambling walk (*pasear*)

strawberry-rhubarb jam

sane living

listening to the radio

"Hi, there."

suds

astonishing colors of rainbow Indian corn

a trip to the North Pole

pampering someone now and then

sanding and shellacking

jingle-bell donkey rides

parents who keep reading the story even after they've noticed that their kid has fallen asleep

having a breezeway

personality profiles

city parks

being someone's pillow

the noise made when you lock the car by remote control

stretching your legs and arms, yawning, and visualizing an ideal day before getting out of bed in the morning

sourdough French toast, dipped in cream-thickened eggs

fresh-cut hay, seasoning in the June sun

Little Women (the 1994 film version)

respecting all living things

shredded toasted coconut

figgy pudding

realizing your strengths

straightening the pantry

hoping that someday you'll cook a steak to perfection

a pub lunch

traveling the information highway

a "memory box"
cats jumping down and walking away
    calmly after being jostled
layering of patterns and colors
a narrow creek spanned by a wooden
    footbridge
a light-up magnifying glass
fraternity rush week
kids' imaginations
firthside and fjordside villages
sand dunes and thickets
the pile of wrapping paper and ribbon left
    after all the gifts have been opened
washable cashmere
a rainy Sunday with your children
langoustines
a secure and refined atmosphere
corrugated green velvet landscapes
homemade dessert
repairable rips
reading a lot of strange books
"Hey Baby, They're Playing Our Song"
    (tune)
frying in bacon drippings
the scent of new-mown hay
snapping towels at people
weekend features in *The Wall Street
    Journal*
jumping to conclusions
blowing bubbles at weddings

anything you have in mind
dumpling soup
intramural basketball
an automobile survival kit
khaki or chino pants
door decorations for each season
face powder
the complete works of Winston Churchill
trapunto stitching through the quilt
    sandwich
fresh batter-fried mushrooms with ranch
    dressing
a coatrack when you need one
the Heisman Trophy
the elegance of a Japanese tea ceremony
something to kick you out of
    unproductive doldrums
contributing something uniquely yours to
    the world
conditioned reflexes
how a branch bends
large, pull-apart rolls
a shake-shingle roof
serving breakfast or snacks to someone
    you love
a set of cotton turtlenecks in a rainbow of
    colors
Marshmallow Peeps, with a shelf life of
    two years
pro-am tournaments

courteous truckers
notary seals
a week-old sparrow
tempera paints
old-time piano stools
sunsets scooped between the dunes
letting your skin breathe
driving along country roads, leaves
    whipping in the wind, through
    woodland valleys that smell of
    the earth
taking someone out for coffee or
    ice cream
hair-flying, shirt-tossing, sun-dripping days
kiss timers
daffodils dancing on fresh clean breezes
heaping sautéed onions on a hot dog
mustache-grooming kits
a row of wooden booths
an Okie from Muskogee
ticketless travel
the squish of wet shoes
a lapel microphone
steaks with A.1. sauce and salt
those who are up and outdoors while the
    day is young and damp with dew
"penny" Valentines, secret love notes, and
    candy hearts
something skimming across the wave of
    your mind

a place to unglob your pen tip

Eastern philosophies brought to the West

brushing out your hair in the sunlight

bib overalls

library books overdue because you are
savoring them

great compotes of honey and crocks of
fresh country butter

abalone hunting

the mother ship

buying T-shirts and shorts on the first
day of spring, then having a blizzard
that night

ice lightly decorating trees

spring onions

gardening tools: rake, hoe, hand fork,
trowel, spade, wheelbarrow, watering
can, seed box, dibble, secateurs,
scissors

gentle light falling through panels of
frosted glass

cluttered rooms

cute one-piece soup bowl and sandwich
plates

the tradition of drinking toasts, from the
old custom of floating toasted bread
in punch

evenings in the recesses of
Paris taxicabs

pictures after parties

saying you're sorry when you hurt
somebody
catching every breeze
children running in and out of narrow
streets like swallows in their chaotic
evening flight patterns
when you see the three dots and know
someone is typing a text message, but
the text has not come through yet
tubs of daffodils and other spring flowers
sweater vests
sea captains' houses
adapting a novel for film
Picardie goblets of tempered glass in
French bistros
incubators
someone's secret summer
hillsides covered by chestnut, lemon, and
olive trees, a wandering shoreline
dotted with mellow hamlets and
splendorous villas
wrapped candies
singing on the school bus
a butler's pantry
canoeing the Yukon
soup ladles
the area between the highway and the exit
lane where cars go when drivers can't
decide what to do next
General Hospital (soap opera)

saying "no" to malls, except maybe once
a year
people who eat corn on the cob in a left-
to-right or "typewriter" style
gleaming light on swift ripples of a lake
square Asian-style plates
hog-calling contests
what we admire in works of art
reveling in the lowbrow
drifting off to sleep
the fuzz on tennis balls
touring glee clubs
one slice of bread spread with peanut
butter slapped against one spread
with strawberry jam
secret handshakes
pop-up baby wipes
early-returning birds
watching model sailboats
a gold-plated megaphone charm dangling
from a dainty chain
buying movie tickets online
argyle socks
plaid shirts
foot powder
lip gloss
the narrative hook
keeping score at a wrestling match
enjoying your vacation
pie at the diner

coupons that would self-destruct after
their expiration date
holiday cookies
early sun rays catching the mountain
summit
being less critical
double knits
when someone invents a faster toaster
the honking of auto horns
when the computer goofs and gives you a
bigger paycheck
really good cheese-and-sausage pizza
the Impressionists (Renoir, Degas, Monet)
pigeons gargling on a fire escape
overlooking the ocean from a candlelit
terrace
glowing all day
plucking tomatoes sun-warm, giving them
a hint of salt and a breath of pepper
inner tubes
My Big Fat Greek Wedding (movie)
unusual-flavored crackers
the Brooklyn Bridge
tactical maneuvers
the 1920s Jazz Age
a sand-between-the-toes walk on the beach
night prowls with flashlights at Halloween
turning off all the lights except those on
the Christmas tree
a round oak table with a single candle

cranberry bogs

ginger ale, saltines, soup

fixed expressions and idioms

polished beechwood against the warmth
of skin

dental insurance

helping a child find unexpected ways of
playing with household objects

when the cake comes out perfect, the
vegetables still have color, the gravy
is smooth, you've used just the right
amount of seasoning, and you feel
pride in your effort

birds crowding the feeder

collecting handbags, supermarket art,
framed cards, Buddha statues,
antique boxes, Art Deco, pictures,
rugs, wooden eggs, matchbooks,
seashells, salt and pepper shakers,
buttons, printer's type, perfume
bottles, labels, copper pennies, quilts

cracking an egg open cleanly with one hand

delicatessens

when you used to visit a seamstress for
hemming and other alterations

store-bought potpourri tucked in a pretty
hankie and cinched with ribbon

windswept moorland

how the things you are happy about
change over time

Greek fishermen's sandals
a lightweight book light
snow-white carpeting
being street-smart
a teasing repartee
buttercups beyond the pasture fence
big, ironed white cloth napkins
mittens in a basket by the back door
a breakfast tray complete with bud vase
      and crossword puzzle
pumpkin bread
double beds
reading ancient wisdom
facial masks
looking irresistible
show-and-tell
following your nose
source code
learning to pot plants
something spellbinding
preheating a Dutch oven in the fireplace,
      then adding bread dough or other
      things to be baked
the days of water beds
Tom Sawyer
fresh, crisp air and sparkling light
inspiring music
a ratified treaty
buying a bunch of anything that is useful
      and nice

asking a beekeeper to let you observe
    honeybees at work
a splinter removed
whitewater rafting
the happiness of heading home
watercolor ombre stripes
the sunny side of an old stone wall
being good-natured
a bright red Oxford shirt
the voice you love to hear
moo goo gai pan
being well-dressed
paying the month's last bill
just a beach, your cat, and the wind
waiting rooms
heat-resistant, clear-glass mugs
Central Park in winter
the mirror in a bar behind the liquor
    bottles that magnifies the effect
armless chairs for the dining table
ranch dressing: buttermilk, sour cream,
    garlic, spices
Anne Morrow Lindbergh's *Gift from the Sea*
the corn being up but not quite in tassel
bright white walls and gaily colored curtains
getting mail
watching Shirley Temple movies
a sunken garden providing sunlight and
    shadow, trees and greenery, stone
    walkways, and a rippling stream

definitions
stereo speakers
watermelon-seed spitting
schematic diagrams
peanut butter and jelly in one jar
saints beloved for their goodness
    and piety
eager beavers
believing in miracles
cowboy boots
seeing the world through each other's eyes
picking cranberries and beach plums
Arizona: tumbleweeds scurrying across
    the desert floor, red-veined copper
    lodes, Scottsdale, cacti
Mother's Day and Father's Day
hairspray artistry
open-faced sandwiches
a brick-paved courtyard with a cluster of
    gift shops
the mysterious writer in a fancy café
eggs hatching
talking to reporters
warm-weather dressing
hide-a-bed sofas
cooling doughnuts hung on long wooden
    dowels
a beehive oven capable of baking many
    loaves of bread at one time
Loch Ness

a plain, thin bracelet
beds of nails
the art of the word
Georgia: brown thrashers singing in the
      pines, sweet scent of Cherokee rose,
      tropical flowers floating in swamps
the call of the coyote
Southern fried chicken and cream gravy,
      hot biscuits, mashed potatoes, a big
      salad, and a huge helping of peas
lakeview bedrooms
da Vinci's codices
Liechtenstein and Uzbekistan, landlocked
      countries surrounded by landlocked
      countries
area codes
always having something to look forward
      to—love, life, work, happiness
children absorbed in quiet play
running through the sand all day
successful cajoling
pink-cheeked faces in knit hats
bundling up for a long walk while the
      turkey is roasting
the bottom of the sundae glass that you
      can't quite reach with your spoon
visiting hours
Native American dream catchers
the frost-flowered surface of a silent lake
unscattered brains

photographers' darkrooms
sleepy people
breadfruit trees
greasing and dusting cake pans
the best waves
the skirling of a bagpipe
escalator steps springing open like an
     alligator's jaw
the sense of promise inherent in the start
     of a new year
days of abstinence
brick cheese
remembering when jeans were only for play
road-test examiners
turning points in life
raw sugar
watching a craftsman whip up a straw hat
the competing claims of nature
pink-and-blue sunsets
menu design
remaining in your comfort zone, health
     zone, and sanity zone
the new car you could win in the shopping
     mall
iced tea served in Mason jars
Loving, New Mexico
the third pancake of a batch being the first
     good one
the quiet days of Indian summer, quiet
     nights of starlight and leaf scuffle

individually wrapped sandwiches
across-the-tub trays
best-case scenarios
a bountiful weekend food table covered
     with an antique lace or linen cloth
     and topped with country pottery, a
     napkin-lined muffin basket, stout
     pitchers for milk or juice, and an
     earthenware vase of wildflowers
companionship
the cardboard core in a toilet tissue roll
losing track of the time
benches under olive trees
scudding clouds of spring
hand-loomed India madras
cuddling your children
hiring help for a party
the next generation
an alpine horn
painting a dream
miniature dachshunds
shivering helping to warm you
exercising at home
the sudden squeal of hidden pigs
making your own happy book
balance beams
two feet of topsoil
sitting on a wooden bridge spanning a
     stream
big red barns

shopping in Hay-on-Wye, the world's
     largest used-book center, on the
     border of England and Wales
"The Lord giveth, the Government taketh
     away."
chunky spaghetti sauce
penicillin
being stranded on a desert island
recalling lines of poetry
the great composers
old farmhouses with tall ceilings
candy
a nor'easter ending
the startling beauty of humble objects
a barn filled with hay, swings, and tunnels
     for hide-and-seek on rainy days
watching Christmas lights twinkling on a
     cabin home
feeling wonderful after washing your hair
slate blackboards
quill pens
rolling lawns and tennis courts
very sharp moonlight
easy-to-use parking meters
a black jacket
electric sanders
foghorns and seagulls
the Holocaust survivors
crafts you make and sell
not smoking

lobster boats coming in under the
     drawbridge
the 6,000 questions of Trivial Pursuit
centrifugal force
breakers so huge that they seem to move
     in slow motion while wind blows
     spray back in gossamer white arcs
     and mists the air with spindrift
Japanese *ma*, the space between
the gentle sounds of a summer Sunday
the scent of wood fires that fills the mind
     with distant memories
secret lands
trunk lunches
roads becoming black velvet ribbons with
     winking frost sequins
being in like Flynn
the habit of making distinctions
"Home Sweet Home"
fondue sets
the bus arriving on time and with empty
     seats
paisleys and toiles
the colony of little indentations on
     a golf ball
the intensity of genius
tinkling china
loudly singing your favorite hymn
freewheeling adventures
a Swiss Army tool on a key ring

spending money on small things: real
    maple syrup, fancy bacon, *Vogue*
    magazine, expensive soaps
mopping up the last trace of gravy with
    the last piece of cornbread
a robot helper for housework
ring-toss rings
the cobalt-blue Mediterranean
V-neck sweaters
buffalo wings in XXX sauce
putting sunscreen on someone
breakfast steak
going someplace you've never been
free makeup samples
learning orienteering
a doll's trousseau
an apology accepted
Swedish cucumber salad with sour cream
romantic fashion looks
requesting a song and dedication from the
    radio station
coffee desserts
lake fish, boiled potatoes, homemade
    coleslaw, fresh-baked bread, and
    cherry pie
your first new car
the helpfulness of a reverse dictionary
a ferret or a pig on a leash
the key to a magic trick
running out after dinner for an ice cream

sable, chinchilla, ermine, mink

being so proud you could burst

the urge to correct all the misspellings on
a menu

feeling cool and serene as a country pond

when suddenly TV dinners didn't come in
aluminum trays, Popsicles didn't have
two sticks, and everything was made
for the microwave

beautiful things, seldom easy

making your house look welcoming on
the outside

Little Red Riding Hood

dogs leaning against your legs

old-time, hard-to-find, bona-fide
lamb's wool dusters

mini Sugar Daddy milk caramel pops

camping cabins

a raisin sauce for baked ham, bubbling on
the stove

fresh flowers at work

finding out you were first on the waiting
list and someone canceled, and so
now you're in!

anything relieving exam-week frustrations

confirmed bachelors

a scar disappearing

making sweet-potato fries

Special Ops

Antigua and Barbuda

the Chatty Cathy doll (1963)
carrying cups of coffee out to the porch to
    enjoy the morning sunshine
a calendar that inspires you
gulls spiraling like paper airplanes against
    the sky
purple cow: grape soda and vanilla ice
    cream
basalt prisms
"knock, knock" jokes
fake ostrich bags
"Where there's a will, there's a way."
pigs-in-a-blanket for dinner
a stack of baseball mitts
just-picked vegetables and fruits
"Soup's on!"
testing for pH
Cheddar-Merlot fondue with apples
glaciers occurring at or near the equator
the tideline
summer love
quilts wrought during long winter
    evenings
finding a place for yourself
a foghorn bellowing
stabbing a block of frozen vegetables to
    make them cook faster
the color and contour of sheets
Alaska: where people go to reinvent
    themselves

math-geek arrogance

tabbouleh and hummus

a noun used as verb

the art of knowing what to overlook

rain barrels

the wonder of life

grinding your own beef

the magnetic/geodetic center of North America

a lifetime warranty

making big root beer floats with long spoons and straws

basically happy people

preparing English-style tea with a teapot, your favorite loose tea, and lemon slices

cuffed Jamaican shorts

a snowshoer in the winter woods

off-peak train fares

short-subject films

brownies with no nuts, crunchy on the outside and gooey on the inside

Colorforms plastic cut-out toy sets

snow shakers

keeping up muscle tone

sweet, hot summer days when terraces were porches and air-conditioning was a pitcherful of lemonade

the blare of a band

being wistful
color schemes for websites
J.J. Audubon's *Birds of America* (book)
entangled rambler roses
T-shirts on backward
visiting your partner's alma mater
spicy chimichangas
finding your own private pleasures
spiral notebooks
settling into a lush green valley to
    dairy-farm
washing a car to make it rain
oil-and-vinegar dressing
houses of cards
oaken floors
a hamburger topped with Béarnaise
responding with a jump of the heart
chicken barbecue with salads, homemade
    breads, and blueberry baked goods
flowers leaning gently on the rims of their
    vases
not resisting truth and beauty
unconventional English
taking care of a friend's child for a
    few hours to give her or him an
    afternoon off
winter as a master miniaturist
the distinctive aroma of garlic or
    bell peppers
your name in hieroglyphics

Tinker Bell in *Peter Pan*

a sidekick who says, "You are correct, sir."

upholding the spirit of the explorer,
      experimenter, inventor

a tapas menu

a grapefruit soufflé

sending someone an article you know will
      be of special interest

true New England chowder: just clams,
      onion, potatoes, and salt pork, served
      with "common" plain, unsalted
      crackers or soda crackers

flashlights with fresh batteries

snuggly nightshirts

the French custom of making a wish each
      time you eat a food for the first time
      in the new year

sod growers

a day for test-drives

a seed that multiplies

blueberries and cream

the saying "dry as a duck"

pewter-colored days

knowing you can go home again

looking closely at the designs of nature

the mind's readiness to make a quick
      connection and then seal it with an
      acrylic topcoat

stirring coffee with your finger

riding the Colorado River on a raft

fake-kidnapping your lover
framed maps
"To thine own self be true."
watching baseball for five hours in
 one day
greeting cards with honeycomb foldouts
a guest who is spiritual and philosophical
leaves to sniff: pennyroyal, dill, bergamot,
 sage, geranium
band marathons
bateau-necked shirts
flour scoops
the voice of a Buddhist monk
a desk built into a wall
bewildered teenagers
curators and docents
lemon wedges for fish
picking flowers for your room at the inn
high IQs
Dolce far niente: It's sweet to do nothing.
getting adequate recognition for a job
 well done
toys and games
vegetable juice
your first rental car
rubber or plastic door runners
if you could wrap every thought in love,
 your life would be transformed
reinventing yourself
a singing vendor

tiddlywinks disks
chafing-dish creations such as veal
   Madeira, beef Stroganoff
embossers that stamp "The Library of ~"
   in books
something suddenly possible
situation comedies
the Super Bowl
your weekend project
taking ghost stories to a clambake
destiny
hams cured the old-fashioned way
financial aid
midnight motorcycle rides
pandemonium
lotions, oils, butters for tanning
playing Clue
walking across the George Washington
   Bridge from New York to New Jersey
   (or vice versa)
asking a child to sing you a song
a wicker chair discovered outside a
   countryside antique store
queries
Noah's soup: two of everything
talking to yourself
the artist within you
hayrack rides
team spirit
napkins soft to the touch

a seasonal collage of pictures of your house
Yale's Whiffenpoofs
step-by-step instructions
the vivid crimson-and-yellow blooms of
    the columbines
reading all the books you never had time for
fabric-covered neckroll pillows, scented
    with a soothing blend of potpourri
spending the morning in bed, watching
    old movies, collaborating on the
    crossword puzzle, making popcorn,
    napping, exchanging long stories of
    childhood, ordering in pizza, and just
    being lazy
new posters for your dorm room
flotation devices
soft robes to settle into
low, burlwood tables
drive-in root beer mugs
the Dick and Jane books
carving sets
"A watched pot never boils."
trouser pockets chortling with change
an over-the-tub whirlpool
drumming of hooves and neighing of horses
spring nights to look forward to
observation and imitation
cherry-and-cranberry cornbread stuffing
microphone-shaped shower soap
taking action

the corded trunk of a sugar maple

melba toast

lentil soup (dal) at the Indian restaurant

the new loaf, warm from the oven

taping a positive message to the bathroom
mirror, refrigerator, and computer
monitor

salt and pepper jars with wire bail tops
and matching vinegar and oil jars
with cork stoppers

the Dr. Zhivago look: tall, furry hat, midi-
length Cossack coat, and boots

sword swallowers

letting children choose the dinner menu
one night a week

the triple kiss, left-right-left

disciples and apostles

crostini with tapenade

a flashlight in your purse

theories of how the universe began

finding something to smile about

snow-capped mountains

feasting on crisp green salads

no-iron clothes

Shetland sheepdogs

showing love for children

shower curtains

an old American appliqué quilt folded at
the foot of the bed

visiting art galleries

feeling deliciously invisible while you
watch the world go by
doggy daycare
bees and hives
candy stores
bright yellow lemons
charming New England villages
beating boredom
throwing the bouquet
shed-style bay windows
the look on a kid's face when watching
magic
the hard-fought decision on what toppings
to order on a pizza
sitting peacefully on a bench
crisp French-fried onions on a burger
acknowledging an astute or insightful
remark
spirituality
idyllic forest settings
buying a sample jar of imported jam
an exit strategy
a bag of chocolate chip cookies
a favorite haunt of the office crowd
flowers for nurturing your soul
shortbread: buttery, crumbling Scottish
biscuit-cake
throwing a surprise party for two
deep and calm feelings
thin pretzels

dolphins, reveling in the buoyant
    pleasures of water
a small picket fence in the snow
idiosyncrasies accepted
monogrammed wine carafes
deep-fried French toast
riding in a hot-air balloon
feeding a parking meter
an Internet café as an "office annex"
hot dogs at the ballpark
watching bakers at work through a
    glass window, pondering turnovers,
    nut breads, doughnuts, and butter
    cookies
a ring around the moon
relishing what you have
rain at night, if you're safe in bed
always growing and thinking up new
    solutions
seasonal businesses
toe space in shoes
French-pressed coffee
gavel-to-gavel coverage
not overreacting
perfect running form
elaborate coats of arms
white Christmas lights
old-timers hanging out in front of the
    firehouse
beautiful beach stones

the lilting song of motion that makes the
    heart rejoice
a great character actor
flower and garden shows
whirring wings
socially responsible investing
getting empathy from your pet
a glass cheese-keeper
The Velveteen Rabbit (children's book)
knee-high nylons
white sauce
sea salt caramel gelato
something sheer as smoke
balloons, banners, hats, noisemakers,
    special invitations, place cards, crepe-
    paper twists, nut cups, and confetti
treasuring private time
blue daisies
learning the zebra is white, with black
    stripes
tricks you use for recalling things
perfect timing
running down dunes
dangling between a past that held a
    different future, and a future that
    would require a different past
kid questions you are prepared to answer
baby leaves
wrought-iron lanterns
getting a tailor to make all your clothes fit

two-tined forks
old white clapboard towns
sitting in chairs on the porch and
    watching the sun
shoeshine boxes
side saddles and horse tack
poached egg on an English muffin
the telescope and its discoveries
learning to be free, willing to take
    reasonable risks, open to others
    and new ideas
cats that eat everything
true beauty being timeless
the last crumpled leaf quivering on the tree
the brain's serendipity
a giant bubble wand
sketching food
whitewashed wainscoting
color: the least expensive and most
    effective decorating touch
visions of dark roast coffee beans, crusty
    loaves, peppery sausage, husks of
    aged Romano and Parmesan cheeses,
    hot Sicilian pizza
cafés with gaily striped umbrellas
candied spearmint leaves
butterscotch-dipped cones
navigating a roundabout
art supply stores
"The Star-Spangled Banner"

mashed potatoes with butter, sour cream,
and chives
knowing all the answers to a game show
while confined to your living room
salt and pepper
the magic of eyeliner
the celebration of being alive
UConn basketball
"In My Life" by the Beatles
Jiminy Cricket
gracious hosts
pages filled with souvenirs and observations
the night-day switch on a rearview mirror
a room decorated in velvet brown,
chrome yellow, caramel tan colors
the way out of a trap being to study the
trap itself: learn how it is built, take it
apart piece by piece
the great elemental sounds of nature:
driving rain, wind in a primeval wood,
and ocean striking the beach
long, low waves
the discovery of a secret view that is
invisible when the foliage is full
the thrill of parades
slowly savoring a soup you made
an emergency bag in the car trunk
a rustic bench in a sequestered spot
wild Maine blueberries heaped onto a
crust and topped with ice cream

the gnomon of a sundial
a miscellaneous category
diet cheaters
thinking of the day, of your home, of your
 family, of things past, of things to come
easy-to-eat finger food
Ken and Barbie's many incarnations
a private walk on a snowy landscape
the slap of a closing book
bells pealing out the good news
oddities like prune or bacon ice cream
sweet faces and hands to wash up before
 supper and kiss before bedtime
Dull Center, Wyoming
what you'd like on your gravestone
being the eyewitness of all you see
the celestial sphere's 88 constellations
carrying a piece of apple pie along with
 a glass of cold milk out to a freshly
 painted deck
herons perched on pilings
crooked cobbled streets
"The privilege of a lifetime is being who
 you are." (Joseph Campbell)
light coming into the soul
scrappy archaeologists
shoelaces that are the perfect length
chenille caterpillars doing push-ups
 through the lawn
an ice-fishing shack

defending your beliefs
nouns
beaver lodges
hill climbing
a quilt on a brass bed
experiencing much love
delicious summer Sunday breakfast
    sandwiches
the patina of old things
the sweet air of spring inspiring a
    different sort of hunger
Mc = Irish, Mac = Scottish
endorsing a candidate
having your talents used but not abused
solving a great mystery
stenciled kitchen cabinets
Shakespeare's seven ages of man: infant,
    schoolboy, lover, soldier, justice,
    pantaloon, second childhood
registering for wedding gifts
catnapping with a cat
the chipmunk lining his winter bedroom
    and stocking his granary
singing in the rain
when, in the middle of a quiet, milder than
    usual night, the melted snow on the
    roof slides off with a thundering crash
a pot of apples, cinnamon sticks, cloves,
    and brown sugar on the way to
    becoming applesauce

half birthdays
everything spelled correctly in the book
     you're reading
an ancient city of Mesopotamia
straight razors
Tabasco sauce
taking your last final of the semester
putting trouble into a boat of leaves and
     sailing it out to sea
decorating magazines
Campbell's green pea soup
pine needles soft as kitten fur
waving out the car's back window
crescent rolls
thick crayons
TV football on mute
French dip au jus sandwiches
supper clubs
sugar cubes
Coney Island hot dogs
barbershop harmonizing
when the color and black ink cartridges
     need to be changed at the same time
scrambled eggs with herbs
creatures with bioluminescence:
     anglerfish, coral shrimp, firefly,
     glowworm, lantern fish, protozoa, sea
     anemone, squid
renting a winter house
looking in all the right places

the *Tonight Show* song
colorful exotic birds
fixing a blown fuse
listening to old rafters, creaky doors, and
loose floorboards
reed organs
a *New Yorker* cartoon on the fridge door
adjusting the car and yourself for good
night vision
a well-worth-it wait
wet suits
ramekins for baked eggs, tiny shrimp, or
chocolate pots au crème
paper sailboats
a "backwards" party—clothes, invitation,
and meal
a mast year, when enormous amounts of
nuts are produced by the trees
the missing last piece of a jigsaw puzzle
the first kiss
at a turn-of-the-century apothecary, a
soda dispensed at an ornate marble
fountain
Thompson seedless grapes
stone gargoyles
having your cat come when you call her
sipping homemade apple cider
viridian glass pitchers
praying in a huge cathedral
the birth of ideas

taking a chairlift up a ski slope to enjoy
    the exhilaration and fresh air
nature walks
having lots of candles burning
the thought of attending culinary school
dropping off a bag of donations for
    Goodwill
nontoxic furnishings
abundant reading time
deep-dish apple pie
the faces of Easter Island statues
hot pulled pork sandwiches
the sensation experienced when an
    elevator stops or takes off too
    suddenly
misty mornings
earth tones
crisped rice
New England's "doughnut belt," south of
    muffin country and north of bagels
garlanding a banister
Hansel and Gretel
potato pancakes, sausages, and
    homemade applesauce
water polo
scheduling your day for peak performance
dew-filled lawns dusted with bairnwort
    and baby's-pet-the-daisy before the
    heads lay in piles of fresh-mown grass
tying up loose ends

Thomas Jefferson: considered by some as
America's first archaeologist
riding a roller coaster
colloquialisms and catchphrases
not taking life that seriously because it's
here to be enjoyed
waffle knit
being alone to talk, to dream, to scheme,
to take aimless drives to no place
special
fresh fruits arranged with a generous
scoop of sherbet
designer jeans and cowboy hats
reminding yourself that everything you
do, think, and dream matters
bobeches around candles to catch
drippings or on chandeliers to hold
suspended glass prisms
a party . . . at someone else's house
high ceilings, beautiful fireplaces, and old-
fashioned molding
having two computer displays
slipping away from shore on a boat
the circling beam from a lighthouse
a tiny plant in a little clay pot
a strange individual you truly adore
surprising your partner and picking
him or her up from work
sunken Spanish galleons
fresh croissants and coffee in bed

wood-smoke smell
almond extract
Where's Waldo?
a blizzard in a snow globe
Senator Robert F. Kennedy
car wax
someone who makes you happy by
    loving you, being alive with you,
    filling up your life
molasses sweet bread
pillow shams
groves of orange and olive trees
gleaming shells in jewel colors, half-
    buried in pearl-white sand
suppertime
Renaissance fairs
sitting down and reading all your old love
    letters
phrenology charts
salt-cured ham steaks
the 240 dots in a Pac-Man game
ditty bags
word clouds
baby dresses
loafers with lug soles
a desktop weather station
cat beer
E-ZPass
Sunday puttering
spice-brown corduroy

ebb tide

street musicians

skinned knees being easier to fix than
broken dreams

delicate fronds

wild black cherry trees

tortellini salad, sliced mozzarella and
prosciutto roll, escargot puffs, and
boeuf en croute

lawn art

your first room at college

Oh, snap!

the crowing of a rooster

orchestra seats

getting up early one warm morning just to
watch the sunrise

the old Chevy

safe sex

lounging around the pool

synchronized clocks

house music

cider mills

a kettle on a wood-burning stove

child-made sailboats on a pond

secret rooms

ladies' night out

Beanie Baby collections

fireflies creating an incredible ballet of
soft light

planning a visit home

a medicine man/shaman
tartlet tins
dirty rice
backyard dining
praying for someone
reading all the books you were assigned
to read in high school and college, but
did not read or did not appreciate
cow chips
an ample supply of local postcards
running your hand along fences or walls
a neck crick disappearing
Brunelleschi's perspective
going to yard sales early on summer days
crisp linen, pink roses, and trays of peaches
crumb crusts
falling asleep while contemplating dinner
tiny cartons of milk
corn snow
deciphering cuneiform or hieroglyphics
a scribe's sanctuary
doggies tumbling into morning, spreading
early birds and careless cats before
them
enough china and silver to serve an army
mustard and soy sauce on a hot dog
sippy cups
a wonderfully desolate beach in November
running a race
a crinkly receipt from a great night out

fabulous online shoe sales

a post office and grocery store being the
only services on the island

boats on the horizon

a natural life, not focused on competition
and achievement

the books on the shelves, a person's
biography

the traffic flow of passed hors d'oeuvres
trays

broiled fish topped by slices of lemon and
cut-up parsley, with browned butter
around it

stacks of old childhood snapshots

mugs of soup

going through a car wash with little kids

the personal assistants of famous people

keeping a foul ball hit into the stands

hot liquid warming you from within

the feel of Ugg fleece on your bare feet

taking advantage of all the opportunities
to keep your mouth shut

a band shell

mini breaks

a wind chime with 100 brass bells

romantic tables for two

sports psychology

watching *Groundhog Day* again, and
again, and again

when the lights flicker but don't go out

fishing for compliments

the quiet in a church before the bride says, "I do"

driving without the radio, CD, or iPod playing

discount tickets

working on your core (abdominals)

people who don't order diet soda at McDonald's

cut flowers at the market

a bay window seat high up around the treetops

making things into doll furniture

finding someone in need and doing something for her or him

a confidante

fields bursting with ripening grain

country inns, castles, old coaching stops

"Silver Bells" (carol)

barbecuing, boiling, baking, broiling, blanching, braising, browning, deep-frying, frying, grilling, slow-cooking, parboiling, poaching, pressure-cooking, roasting, stewing, sautéing, simmering, steaming, toasting

a species coming off the endangered list

curling irons

how to throw a screwball

collecting books of lists

the warmth of a tumble-dried shirt

having breakfast by the window on the
    occasion of a child's first snowfall
"I'd Rather Be Reading."
July afternoons roaring and rumbling with
    thunderstorms
discovering a great junk store
the Zen of snow removal
democracy
swimming with a kickboard
a basket of tender, flaky, fresh-from-the-
    oven biscuits
strawberry ice-cream shortcake
heavy teak deck chairs
feeling lucky to be born a human
cleaning out your emotional closet
open exhibits at a museum
reaching out to people
roll-back cuffs
notebooks with blank pages to be filled
a white-gold sunrise
carpenters' plans
blue Wedgwood china
Pennsylvania and Swiss chocolate
understanding that for more than
    99 percent of human existence, life
    was enormously different from today
dressing a scarecrow
laissez-faire
frost-touched streets
therapy that heals

a concept album
cotton clothing
longing for certain happinesses
baking a crock of beans overnight
the point on a mammal's back where it
    cannot reach to scratch
a hoedown
a pencil reading along with
    every word it writes
choosing a tennis racket
kitchen stools
a day away from your computer
Le Creuset cookware
painkillers
Prince Edward Island wool caps
the science of everyday life
jovial fellows
the best-kept romantic secrets
mountains of produce
watching the moon at night and finding
    out why it looks the way it does
polished copper
taking down badminton or volleyball nets
women who dress for aerobics class in
    dangling earrings, coordinated outfits,
    and full makeup
chewable vitamins
the wind chimes that have hung in front
    of your house for years, in all types of
    weather

smoke detectors

sharing a dream

moving far north

mountain-ledge flowers blooming on
sky-high rocky peaks

real friends who ask thoughtful
questions

pickled onions

when something strikes a spark of
interest, following it

peaked roofs

having a private picnic

Popsicle sticks

the greatest truths being the simplest

Belgian lace curtains

master sommeliers

cardiovascular fitness

New York's Finger Lakes

zeroing in on a solution to a problem

near-perfect weather

a banana clip for hair

photos of regular moments, the going-
through of everyday motions, the
quiet moments

Earth from outer space

clay-potted English ivy

numbers committed to memory

eating all your snack bar items before the
movie even starts

unclogging a toilet

places that have more sun than cloudiness
Acheulian hand axes from the Lower
    Paleolithic period
the Library of Congress
bucktoothed kids
the company of a mountain
sunken treasure
a hotchpotch of scenery
riding well-schooled ponies through
    woods and on the hillsides
parking lights
dawn shimmering with dew, sunrise on
    lawn and meadow
being praised in class
glass beads
things that are part of our dreams and hopes
soft cowl-neck pullovers
the difference between New England and
    Manhattan clam chowder
planting a beach umbrella
snow on your eyelashes
winter fruit
eau de toilette
great elm trees
large-item trash pickup day
using a pumice stone
lemon to keep vegetables and fruits from
    turning brown
Puss in Boots
pretzel nuggets

the whisk-broom sound of footsteps on
   fallen leaves
a new adventure every day
seeing objects formed by clouds
the rope on fancy restaurant menus
hearing your teenager say, "I love you,
   Mom."
sitting in a cozy booth
a butter slicer with wire dividers
"If I Loved You" (song from the play and
   movie *Carousel*)
a patient mother who does not get
   annoyed by things that don't actually
   matter
buttered or cream-cheesed date bread
recovering from a big disappointment
decorating in "early college" or "early
   married"
fish-watching with polarized glasses
bees playing on small kazoos
a pajama day
"The Sugar Plum Tree" (poem)
moving to a new house
shops where individuality shines
white-tailed deer in the clearing
remembered tales beside a fire
curved park benches
a restaurant where guests cook their own
   steaks, lobsters, and shrimp on a
   table grill

soda fountain memories you'll never lose

a catnip-filled sock

geologic marvels like the Grand Canyon
and the Himalayas

playing the *Nutcracker Suite* at Christmas
dinner

silvery milkweed pods opening

platters of good things to eat

a breeze tiptoeing into the room, afraid to
intrude

babushkas

blue waters, white sails, and ruddy
swimmers

me time

a vast wonderland of soaring, snow-capped
peaks, turquoise lakes, glittering
glaciers, and tumbling waterfalls—
all framed by dense green forests

Michigan City, Indiana

kitchen windows

a tray of scones and pot of honey

no sound except the branches clicking
together and a vast, far skein of wind
flung down from the sky

truck stops and little country towns off
the freeway

your adrenaline starting to pump at the
thought of leaving work and going
home

climbing atop an observation tower

abacus beads
latte art
the wild blue yonder
lean meat
the filibuster in *Mr. Smith Goes to
     Washington* (movie)
a Technicolor sunset
a good Monday
babies who never cry
buying your first home
grapefruit, sliced bananas, berries,
     cornflakes, and poached eggs for
     breakfast
lovely ghostly zings that a guitarist's
     fingers make
cooking for people all weekend
a cherished memory
the social role-playing of clothing
cheerfulness
jewel necklines
Baby Boom (movie)
learning HTML
reading between the lines
no expiration date
cozy bed jackets
consuming M&M's by color groups
antique Chinese porcelain covered bowls
     for sugar or candy
a pot of tea produced when anything
     momentous occurs

the superior taste of food cooked over a
    charcoal fire
Pepe's Pizzeria in New Haven,
    Connecticut
hidden windows
a riot of colors
the wheezing of an accordion
a draftsman's tool kit
deciding on favorite Super Bowl
    commercials
hours spent organizing and cleaning
big baskets for magazines or yarn
terra-cotta freckles
a menu with all the words spelled correctly
the wonder of the circulatory system
teaching within the home
a milky white nub of sand amid the
    cyan sea
recycling old mobile phones and
    eyeglasses
photosynthesis
gumball dispensers
good afternoons
rainstorms
bike riding along the Potomac River
autumn bonfires of gathered twigs
the texture of pudding
when you are on a road that you do not
    know and there's a driveway to turn
    around in unobtrusively

sensing when something is different but
    not being able to put your finger on
    precisely what it is
dinners that include a green salad and
    French bread with butter
cabin lights
a first edition of a book
worth-it restaurant food
writing a poem
never dramatizing a difficulty
maple cream cheese spread
coal shoveling
short-sleeved camp shirts
poachette rings for eggs
really thick, special or insightful, thought-
    provoking books
a mixum-gatherum
would-be artists
building a bed frame
fashion shows
making sure the water from the shower
    hits the back of your neck
Arctic cloudberry jam
dime novels
the dressed-in-black student set, often artsy
hand-me-downs
the exhilaration of cleaning out, throwing
    away, giving away, and selling—
    opening up some space and
    breathing room

classroom instruction
using the sandwich plates
a wire caddy for paper cups, ketchup,
    mustard, pickles for picnics
old-fashioned square dances
warm sun and sea spray
interstate highways
Apollo space missions
carrot tops
new cookbooks
the body's first surge of energy in the
    morning
an absence of billboards
"Attention means attention." (Zen saying)
the brisk dusk of a late October evening
washing your hands before you eat
the whole day on skis, with a picnic lunch
lipstick in tiny plastic tubes
baked ziti
the delicate content of recipes
staging a children's vehicle parade with
    scooters, bicycles, and skateboards
    festooned with crepe paper
the delights of finding first spring flowers
finishing a long-overdue project
sidewalk cafés
cedar-stump furniture
the scientific method
water bottles
shower gifts

Pikes Peak
family time
listening to a complete recording of an
    opera prior to attending it
climbing up on a hill at sunrise
fizzy science experiments
staying home on New Year's Eve
the feeling you get around five o'clock in
    the afternoon, after realizing you've
    accomplished a lot
having a pantry
reaching for the sky
the details in a slice of radish
water crackers
sandbags when you need them
an egret in your backyard
large, framed pieces of seascapes,
    landscapes
escaping the winter blahs
jean jackets
major kitchen appliances
kits: cosmetic, dopp, first aid, medical,
    mending, sewing, shoeshine, tackle,
    toilet, tool, travel
intensity and abandon
roll-neck sweaters
red clover, sugar maples, hermit thrushes,
    and honeybees
loaded baked potato soup
bacon and pork sausages

planning a weekend of doing something
you usually tell yourself you're too
unadventurous for

scaling down your wants

splurging on a midweek dinner out

the tons of things that kids do better
than adults

expanding your horizons

double-bagging the groceries

using vine-ripened sweet summer
tomatoes to make tomato sauce and
freeze it for winter

ambient music creating an atmosphere

mentally preparing yourself for a big
change

eating alone

poaching fruit for compotes

motion-activated lights

playing poker

thinking caps

picking the perfect nacho off someone
else's plate

the feel of a whirlpool

miniature artichokes

catching a fish bare-handed

Wynken, Blynken, and Nod

panoramic murals

throwing away half of the papers in
your files

staying on the fringe of politics

types of beds: baby, brass, bunk, canopy,
    crib, cot, davenport, double, feather,
    hammock, Hollywood, hospital, iron,
    king-size, Murphy, queen-size, roll-
    away, round, single, trundle, twin,
    vibrating, wall, water
summer camp: learning how to make
    belts, gimp lanyards, put on skits
college meal plans
creating a snow sculpture
classes with chairs in a circle
hanging the tinsel
bacon, lettuce, tomato, and avocado
    sandwiches
individual soufflé dishes
the last few answers of a crossword
    puzzle
honest signs, like "Road Repairs—
    Next 12 Years"
curling your hair
the silence that pervades a crowded
    elevator when the doors close
poker parties
Greek foods
weather brewing
peanut-butter makers
a portrait in the snow
taco dinners
succeeding in not raising your voice
    during a fight

lavish buffet spreads
a day with no interruptions at work
farm markets with the best fresh milk
someone who "has your back"
pulling all-nighters before exams
trompe l'oeil insouciance
crystal chimes
a street full of bookstores and galleries
keeping your secrets
walking around a swimming pool
erasers that work well
morning dew
She sells seashells by the
    seashore. (tongue twister)
remembering when there were no movie
    ratings
an aromatic puff of frying onion wafting
    out the door
canaries singing more when they have
    company
free admission
stratocumulus, cumulus, and
    cumulonimbus clouds
a Sunday night salad bowl
group traveling
a bed of clams
floats in a parade
tying your hair back
orchard maps
the tea table

the satisfaction of lifting your own
    homemade waffles out of a steaming
    waffle iron
converting a toolshed into a studio
Utah: Salt Lake, Bryce Canyon, clean,
    wide streets, choir, honeybees
the receptionist at your gym
pieces-of-eight
human nervous system messages being
    transmitted at about 180 to 200 mph
ducks water-skiing to a halt
receiving forgiveness
jazzercise
syllabub
birches that look like paintbrushes whose
    tips have been dipped in rouge
the 1768 edition of the *Encyclopaedia
    Britannica*
a firm handshake
having your coffee in the park
two shakes of a lamb's tail
the fine red and blue threads running
    through new dollar bills
taverns in the colonial era
Milky Way candy bars
the taiga, the tundra, and the alpine
    regions of Denali
playing Old Mill
once-a-year headaches
the order in which you open the mail

weaving cat's cradles and other string
  figures
headstrong people
a yoga/exercise space in your house
sailing half-dazed through the air on a
  swing suspended from a tree
West Virginia: twin panhandles, Harpers
  Ferry, the Potomac, the Greenbrier
sand-sifting
grilled meat served with salty French fries
Skippy peanut butter
listening to classical music during lunch
yellow wax beans
soy candles
give-and-take in a relationship
corn custard
tennis on TV
creamed turkey
pistachio nuts
the best cheerleaders
bursting into song
milk

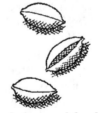

delectable creations made hot and fresh
  every morning
a lovely villa with charming hosts
choosing, at whim, quiet back roads
Phillips Exeter Academy
the pattern in which a brick wall is laid
responding wittily
the peeling of a Polaroid snapshot

keeping a fire burning as a welcome
fingerling potatoes
informing TV characters of impending
    danger, thinking that they can hear you
ham and Cumberland sauce
a toe-wiggling, breeze-blowing day
negotiating with a genie
ribbon dancing
getting the answer you want from the
    Magic 8-Ball
pre-sliced cheese
the courage to adopt children
writing themes
sowing seeds evenly
dotting your *i*'s with smiley faces
plump floor cushions
wine lists in fat binders
the smell of grilled onions in Grand
    Central Terminal
courteousness
a strolling trio of musicians
army buddies
O, the oldest letter in the alphabet
moving hurdles
when the lakes are high
red-checked tablecloths
insulated window shades
cocoa butter soap
buying an I-feel-good hat and wearing it
    on your better days

quiet places: a garden, a reading room in
    a library, a corner nook in a café, a
    botanical garden, a chapel, a rotunda
    at a museum, a closet, a hammock
learning to make the perfect cup of coffee
rain-sensitive windshield wipers
sailing a felucca down the Nile at night
Internet access exactly when you need it
zingy burritos
a cakewalk
cable television
a charismatic figure
calling in sick when you are sick
making clothes
home, where we tie one end of the thread
    of life
spotting a celebrity
a romp in the hayloft
bamboo torches
the Chicago Blackhawks hockey team
denim belts
full-spectrum lightbulbs simulating
    sunlight
medallions Béarnaise
a chance to recognize and celebrate
    someone you love dearly
REM sleep
savoring cool summer mornings to relax
    and energize
springing along a sidewalk

opening the car window and resting your
    forearm on the door
crayons without their "papers"
catching someone smiling to himself or
    herself
an elevator's "ding!"
Christmas chains to count the days
marquetry floors
the evolving collage of your daily life
time to browse
the look of a room after you clean it
dusting off the camera
watching a sushi chef prepare nigiri
a ladybug kicking her six feet in a tantrum
the true meaning of an object, seen only
    with reference to its relationships,
    its context
bartering for fun
picnic scenes
robins' eggs
being quietly sexy
a well-crafted chair
remembering people's names long after
    they've forgotten yours
the Indianapolis 500
bobby socks
someone to miss
Scrat, the obsessive rodent with a
    Sisyphean pursuit of an acorn in the
    Ice Age movies

hanging pans
getting the first appointment of the day
maple butternut squash
a painters' or writers' workshop on Block
    Island, Rhode Island
rolling up your sleeves
Little League baseball
old newspaper clippings
Martha Graham dance pieces
cooking oil spreading out in a skillet
postage stamps: first introduced in Belgium
a heap of homemade French fries
volunteering to help out in a soup kitchen
"Keep a thing for seven years and you'll
    find a use for it." (proverb)
a waiters' race
someone calling to check on you when
    you're sick
passing the bar exam
spinning quite a yarn
the sea's bioluminescence
favorite dorky shoes
mime artists
staying out of courtrooms
ballroom dancing
the Hoover Dam lit at night
living in the woods near the edge of a lake
medical research
polliwogs
having an "art stash"

taking a food-and-drink dictionary to
a restaurant
milkweed pods ripening and freeing
their seeds to sail away on fluffy
parachutes
possibilities for refreshment and
discovery
the smell of Band-Aids
solo, duo, trio, quartet, quintet, sextet,
septet, octet, nonet, dectet
the hoot of an owl
wading pools
getting along well with others
a bean bursting noiselessly through the
mold in the garden
eating at the boat dock
fluffy pillows
grilling over slow coals
leaving a used book somewhere for
someone else to happily discover it
Canada geese returning in long, dark
distant lines
ham and apple butter on a croissant
the sacred city of Lhasa, Tibet
skeins of yarn
floor plans
the poem "June" by James Russell Lowell
doors that open amiably to dogs
shambling home
bowls filled only with yellow M&M's

beaming parents of the new graduate

things advertised that are actually in stock

different camouflage patterns

slowing down, deep looking

miniature ballotins from Godiva

the rings of circus acts

listening to the sound of your own
    breathing

entering a baseball park through turnstiles

coming home from work exhausted but
    fulfilled

finding the perfect adjective in a
    thesaurus

escaping from an overwhelming
    department store and buying an
    armful of flowers from the vendor on
    the corner

a spider's web of streets

the silence of a leafless landscape

Ruffles potato chips

things Mother never told you

homemade maple syrup, real cream, real
    butter, and heated plates

church suppers

being classy

the unwrapped gifts of nature

burying yourself in a pile of magazines
    you seldom have time for

the indentations on the side of a
    dictionary

cardigan sweaters
the best information
cast-iron and brass beds
turkey legs
potato mashers
falling in love with the summer lifeguard
dollhouses and plastic furniture
a white-fence-enclosed rose garden
curling and uncurling your toes
boutique farming
clipping box bushes into perfect spheres
the pattern on a dress your mother wore
a whisper impossible to resist
international road signs
good children on a plane
inviting your best friend over and giving
      each other manicures and new
      hairstyles
forgiving someone
extra-long loaves of bread spread with
      softened butter
luxuriating in how an author uses words
a properly exposed low-light photograph
improving steadily
the name "Keir Brian"
encaustic painting
rimless eyeglasses
a lucky penny in a bottle
handwritten letters that include photos,
      cartoons, dried flowers, or quotations

colored markers

votives flickering on windowsills in
defiance of the darkness

making a balloon dog

fake fur coats

cycling derbies

hodgepodges

the paper stretched across the examining
table at a doctor's office

leafy suburban campuses

ventriloquists' dummies

a harpist playing at a buffet extravaganza

being a night person

learning how to live well with others

having the backup files when your
computer crashes

red: beets, radishes, red cabbage,
tomatoes, cherries, red plums,
strawberries, cayenne, cloves

writing an advertisement

side pouches on furniture for magazines

sliced pound cake with butterscotch
sauce

art as therapy

kissing potions

courage and conviction

combining different cereals

zoris, Asian sandals with wooden
bottoms

Italian suits and collarless shirts

Texas toast: thick slices of white bread
brushed with butter and grilled
the mesmerizing flames of a roaring fire
taco salad of mixed greens, cheese, taco
meat, tomato, and jalapeños in a
crunchy shell
the silent industry of chlorophyll
bringing home the bacon
setting an old chair or rocker out in the
garden
being free-spirited
an hour or two fly-fishing in a quiet pool
the language spoken by fast-food
restaurant employees
rail-splitting contests
the coldness of the freezer aisle
hot sun cooled by a sea breeze carrying
the heady scents of pine trees and
clam flats
the Duchenne smile: when two different
facial muscles fire, forming a genuine
smile
the first meal you cook in your first
apartment
kayaking among dozens of tiny islands
urban legends
perihelion, when we are closest to the Sun
touch-and-guess exhibits
Arby's Beef 'n Cheddar sandwich with
Arby's sauce

when someone you love tells you he or
     she misses you
paper plates
the fresh green of spring's young shoots
walking faster than cars sitting in traffic
a balloon flying to freedom
the cotton-maker's symbol
chevron stripes
muumuus
two old people sitting on lawn chairs on
     the driveway of their house or condo
a large plump rabbit loping by
gargantuan slabs of meat
big gestures
10-gallon hats
the first time you held hands
middle-school graduation
calm weather
making a wish on an eyelash
pieces of willowware
eating in the kitchen
the 14 meridians or energy pathways in
     the body
a clipper ship captain's desk with slanted
     lift lid and drawers on the sides
escorts offering their arm
having a briefcase in third grade
jade-colored lagoons
a vacant seat next to you on an
     international flight

splurging on a spectacular party
alternating the books you're reading
falling in love
llama or pony trekking
kicking through the goalposts
a babysitter when you need one
a neat way to dispose of bacon grease
a pride of lions
homographs, words spelled alike but
    with different meanings
bagless vacuum cleaners
a teacher on summer vacation
muttering under your breath
unarguable fundamentals
the ticking of an old clock
people who answer your emails
uncrinkled aluminum foil
falling asleep when the plane takes off
    and waking up when it lands
changing habits
surprise birthday parties
library reading rooms
the certain way you smile at each other as
    soon as your eyes meet
hot sauce "chugging"
improbabilities in TV shows and movies
day trips for empty-nesters
baths in the dark, with candles lit at the
    last minute
saddle soap

kneading dough
soft-shell clams and crabs
writing a bestselling book
green grass and the smell of it
the Sugarplum Fairy
thin Swedish roll-up pancakes served with
    lingonberries or blueberries
the *Beany and Cecil* cartoon
sailboat sails
asterisms, clusters of stars or any six-
    rayed star-shaped figure seen in some
    crystal structures under reflected or
    transmitted light
"A musician must make music, an artist
    must paint, a poet must write, if he
    is to be ultimately at peace with
    himself." (Abraham Maslow)
getting an early start
oceanfront dining rooms
Eastman Lake, New Hampshire
familiar sounds of the Deep South
body elements: aluminum, arsenic,
    calcium, carbon, chlorine, cobalt,
    copper, fluorine, hydrogen, iodine,
    iron, magnesium, manganese,
    nitrogen, oxygen, phosphorus,
    potassium, silicon, sodium, sulfur,
    zinc
wraparound corner windows
the cool feel of a metallic necklace

children with a strong work ethic

walking a mile in another person's shoes

practicing basketball at a park

seeing each thing as new

figuring out "affect" and "effect"

belt-in-the-back coats

using a word like *fingerbreadth*

grandmothers who put olive oil in their
hair

ice cream served in metal stemmed dishes
that get all frosty on the outside

the part of the envelope that tells where
to place the stamp as if you couldn't
figure it out

reducing the number of times you feel
overwhelmed

holding your tummy in

driving against the arrow in a parking lot

old-fashioned straw dispensers

in-line skating

cooling off at the pool

a rotating toaster or gridiron that lets
toast and meat cook evenly on all
sides without being handled

pogo sticks

Heinz 57 tomato ketchup

warm water on a cold face

insulated windbreakers

snapping turtles hibernating side by side
on the pond bottom

the penciled flights of departing geese
scrawled against the sky

watching the sunset and the world turning
backward

Valentine candy hearts

Busch Gardens season passes

common sense

the sign for your exit

"What is essential is invisible to the eye."
(*The Little Prince*)

trying to answer the phone before the
answering machine picks up

peaceful countryside

appreciating when the ATM gives you
money and your card

a beautifully bound book

Scandinavia's climate

bicycle paths among the sand dunes

French-speaking Belgians

people on a sidewalk watching TV in a
store window

messy piles of shoes in the closet

great-grandmother's cameo

knowing how good you have it

monarch butterflies

walk, trot, and canter gaits

agreeableness

pork chop weather, when dinner needs to
be heavy-duty

the friend who introduced you to Mr. Right

Sting and The Police
warm-weather lunch hours
brand-new notebooks
Virginia country ham served over cornbread
    and covered with maple syrup
the last appointment of the day
a pond that freezes into a natural
    ice-skating rink
shrimp-shaped earrings
refinishing a flea-market find
when homework assignments get lighter
    toward the end of the year
breaking horses in Montana
making a beeline
family-style all-you-can-eat restaurants
manhole covers
a T-bone's filet and sirloin
the setting sun splashing a pink tinge
    over fleecy clouds
realizing you have more time to get
    things done than you thought
a tearful tune
small salads
a bag of lemons
being secretly relieved
distance learning
Humpty Dumpty
England's Houses of Parliament
What's Up, Doc? (movie)
stain-resistant fabrics

helping someone do laundry
sliced ham with mustard pickles
planting by the moon
music for ballet practice
pizza cutters
stopping being a perfectionist
outfitting a new car
the daily mail
a truck stop with great spicy ribs and
    sweet-potato pie
knowing the absolute right way to do
    something
fresh pink tablecloths and huge pink
    cotton napkins
chicken-fried steak and country gravy
kitties licking
a toe loop in ice-skating
creating a signature dish
a watermelon stabbed with a knife so that
    the rind splits with a crackle and the
    smell comes pouring out
laughter being the best medicine
doing the dishes right after dinner
deep country
an antique red hand-stenciled wooden
    sled with dark pine runners
automobile brochures
an intensive, eleventh-hour effort to
    accomplish or finish something
    before a deadline

the letter *W*'s three syllables
slot-car races
the pile of stuff you have cut out and saved
slim, crustless sandwiches
returning to your warm and comfy bed
 after using the bathroom in the
 middle of the night
sneakers' crisscrossed laces
charm school
magnetic poetry or Mad Libs
lending out your snowblower
the verdant countryside
"Knowledge is power."
doing well on the back nine
what lies beyond the stars
a day when you do not swear
stopping at "enough"
the unhurriedness of brunch
strange, unintelligible symbols for washing
 instructions on clothing labels
going to the edge rather than staying
 stuck in the middle
lion taming
animals and toys for a nursery
scented shoe pillows
the purpose of all those lines and
 markings on a gym floor
French onion soup served in a giant
 Vidalia onion
great shadows lengthening in the fields

rare-book collecting
Snap-on Tools trucks
rain lovers
Internet Movie Database (IMDb)
garlic bread
firing on all four cylinders
drifting down France's beautiful Canal du
    Midi on a hotel barge
a book of codes
whittling wood
reflections on wet pavement
watching someone shave or shampoo
not burping at the dinner table
something springing from mind's eye, to
    sketch pad, to reality
eyes that never tell lies
ship's clocks
the Monday wash
a child's wisdom
root beer and spaghetti
grass-sledding
seeing happy parents
doing the right thing even when no one is
    looking
time for cozy dinners of soup and bread
    and indoor games by a toasty fire
flats of pansies
mist over the rolling meadows drifting away
sending small whimsical gifts to brighten
    a long day

trimming logs for cabin building

wildlife preservation

"bowl" haircuts

deep carpeting

children punctual for a meal they love

the first video game you ever played

a Rhode Island barrel clambake, including
scalloped oysters

a camp breakfast

blue-jeaned students

sizing up the options and choosing well

getting out of the got-to-tell-all, lay-it-on-
the-line syndrome and remembering
how nice it is to have a secret

knowing how to change a tire

when hiking through snow, using the
footsteps of one who has boldly gone
before you

positive daydreaming

gray T-shirts

picking up things with your toes

refusing to acknowledge that your
shortcut is not actually shorter than
the other route

the natural connection of events

that feeling you get when you walk into a
quiet church

taking a cooking course in Paris

trying to explain why something is a
favorite of yours

shopping at garage sales

spontaneous originality in communication

rollaway beds

large textual databases

a 30th birthday

patenting your invention

a place to stretch out on the sand, to
beachcomb for unusual driftwood
formations

pima cotton shirts

the long walk up the aisle at the end of
a movie

football towers

tongs

Down Under

redrawing your view of the world with
visualization

victory over incompetence

being spry

J.R. Ewing

lunch served poolside

unbelievably tender filet mignon

cleaning windshields

suiting up

a "blooming onion" and horseradish dip

an archaeological dig

a scintilla

children's eyes

crossing something dreaded off a list of
things to do

banging screen doors
buying a book and getting lost in a
     new topic
feeling satisfied with the rightness of the
     present moment
vacuum bottle holders with straps
seed catalogs starting to arrive in the mail
enjoying popcorn, songs, and campfire
     camaraderie
learning to service your own car
"Roger, Wilco"
spacing out
elite troops
bread ovens
being brave
telephoning overseas
a tiny restaurant that specializes in
     lunches and afternoon tea
anonymity
baby bird time
father's den or man cave
plastic bags that zipper shut
garam masala
power tools
just deserts
The Moon-Spinners (movie)
the 100,000 religions that anthropologists
     estimate have existed
not having to pick up wet towels
a wonderful art exhibit just a taxi ride away

seating that is girl-boy-girl-boy
a trophy for being a participant
handbag design
bleached sand dollars
drying flowers
chefs cooking food on hibachi grills
    with flair and charisma
snap (kisslock) purses
impulse buying
frosty nights and blue-sky days
disco music
vocalisms like *um, uh, er, ew, huh*
steep-sided fluted brioche, the richest,
    butteriest, and airiest of all breads
a time for all things
toga parties
pedal-pusher pants
icicle-style Christmas lights
writing in a beautiful hand
negotiating a traffic circle/rotary
seeing others enjoying something
    you created
a lost pet reunited with its owner
cooling swims
salad with oil and vinegar and fresh,
    hot French bread
the kangaroo, koala, and wombat
an old warehouse restaurant with
    stained-glass windows
solids-and-stripes billiards

sad, romantic, nostalgic, wistful, peeved,
    kittenish feelings
wild turkeys
African violets
serving Chinese takeout in bento boxes
cloak-and-dagger operations
officiating with confidence
keeping your own commonplace book
art or stock portfolios
a warm May day
childhood report cards and art projects,
    high school yearbooks, photo albums,
    diaries, and love letters
plastic ponchos in bright colors
listening to the news
pegged coatracks
bar cookies
"When I'm good, I'm very good; but when
    I'm bad, I'm better." (Mae West)
the yellow-orange blooms of the daisy-like
    black-eyed Susan
rough wood
a butterfly flying into you
working on a bibliography
advertising in the Yellow Pages
assembling for a rehearsal
hearing "your song"
open restaurant kitchens
the crunch of sugar snap peas
rainbow cakes

chopsticks-only dining
fifty-two promising weeks
a long-lasting lightbulb
machine-washable things
sharing in the planning, shopping, and
cooking of a dinner party
a baby squirrel
penuche icing on spice cake
magical winter places
dialogue and negotiation
seltzer bottles
camp stoves
looking 50 when you are 60
the detour signs actually taking
you back to the right road
the days of miniskirts
honey mustard pretzels
someone's silent thoughts
roasted green peppers stuffed with a
pungent meat-and-rice filling, dressed
in tomato sauce and cheese
tending to your knitting
Sheetrock
church spires
Thanksgiving, when there may be a brush
of snow on the ground and a hint of
frost in the air
cheetah cubs
smooth renovations
cable car rides

the corners of your mind
crabmeat-filled mushrooms
being all alone with a black-and-white
    movie on television and a comfy pair
    of pajamas, cutting and pasting
    a scrapbook
Tweety Bird
ice cubes tinkling like wind chimes
platypuses in Australia
being forgiven
Julia Roberts, actress, and her smile
a swaying sea of grass
oval, pear, marquise, and emerald
    diamonds
parents eating hot lunch with their
    children once a year
potatoes Anna: a crisp hunk of potato
    heaven served with sour cream
    and chives
the Gerber baby
baked beans cooked in maple syrup and
    mustard
seeking out uncrowded stretches of beach
clotted cream the rich color of yellow
    garden roses
October: the month to exhale the hot,
    stuffy laziness of summer and inhale
    the cool, brisk life of fall
framing a favorite recipe
retiring on your own terms

the ease with which we fall in love or fall
    in love all over again
writing letters in an outdoor café
theories on pyramid building
Stonehenge at twilight
marinating on an idea
1961
being wonderfully alone on a frozen
    country pond
the universe
the song of the mower
being happy as a clam
periwinkle shells
making a fall clothes-buying list
    each year
barbed wire
foliage tours
a rooster weathervane
Gnaw Bone, Indiana
"as quick as a wink"
an even keel
a grace period
responding to a challenge
a culinarian
"When in doubt tell the truth." (Mark
    Twain)
Aladdin and his Wonderful Lamp
eating soup after pig-out weekends
buying and painting unfinished furniture
sneakers with dress suits

the sound of a clock ticking, and nothing
    else
mutual funds
going all out
Nordic skiing
glabella: the space between your forehead
    and eyebrows
county fair signs
someone with the biggest smile in
    the world
resting under a favorite tree
buttery Danish dough
honeymoon spots
being yourself
Mozilla Firefox
your signature
crimped hair
an escape hatch
Cracker Jacks
twilight hour
McDonald's hot caramel sundaes
Oxford, England
eggdrop soup
playing *Jeopardy!*
booster rockets
the furling and unfurling of leaves
the shudder of pipes in the morning
acoustic guitars
listening to the tinkle of Taiwan bamboo
    wind chimes

361

the luxury of a fresh towel
noise-free zones
candies under pillows
sable watercolor brushes
Plan B
bicycling in the evening
open rolling fields and stone walls
shivaree serenades for newlyweds
barbecue pits
backup vocalists
fanning yourself
balconies overlooking a brook and forest
two-handed backhands
uncovering an unexpected patch of
    wildflowers
user submissions
using a self-discovery workbook
a newsroom at deadline
plastic wrap that cooperates
coming up with ideas
when you have amazing tolerance with
    something that previously you have
    had little or no tolerance for
khaki walking shorts
synchronization of noises
"The most beautiful thing we can
    experience is the mysterious."
    (Albert Einstein)
a neat twist of fate
collectible enamelware

the combination of fall colors and
    waterside atmosphere
good broth
blooming tropical flowers
Burberry's nova check
the importance of secret places—
    a neighbor's attic, a forgotten gazebo,
    a closed door and a comfortable chair
cutting open a grapefruit and finding a
    sprouted seed
having an unfortunate knack for
    approaching a set of double doors
    and always pushing the locked one
desires made out of nostalgia and
    imagination
network sports introductory music
mountain vistas
one's modus vivendi
Cardini's original list of six ingredients for
    Caesar salad: romaine lettuce, garlic,
    olive oil, croutons, Parmesan cheese,
    and Worcestershire sauce
standing in the doorway, embracing
    sheets brought in from the line with
    an end-of-summer smell in them
Trekkie or trekker?
finding a pair of never-worn shoes in the
    back of your closet
a great green mound of moss
well-filled bookshelves

"Hush-a-bye, Baby" (lullabye)

outdoor careers

strands of wood, mother-of-pearl, shell, yellow jade, and coffee bean beads

chopping fresh herbs

snow on the side of the road

who'd-a-thunk anecdotes

a rousing rendition of the "Hallelujah Chorus"

bus excursions

lame ducks

bakery boxes tied with string

summertime

wiggling your flip-flops over the edge of the porch

playing "spy" in the woods

trials and tribulations

remembering Father paying $4 for a full tank of gas

babies in bootees and snow overalls

parasailing in the Andes

freestanding full-size mirrors

The Pledge of Allegiance

a smiling countenance

beaches you're sure no one else has discovered

rekindling friendships

the *Titanic*, the only ocean liner sunk by an iceberg

Revolutionary and Civil War reenactments

empanadas

the honk of car horns and car alarm
    systems

hanging balloons in the windows

butcher-block tables

retirees in the Sunbelt

hearing your child sing a solo on stage

eating six hot dogs and drinking five
    Cokes at a picnic

whisper-soft, lacy-knit afghans

raccoons and squirrels scampering in
    the bush

never having used training wheels

Winnie-the-Pooh's chuckle

a single flower meaning more than a dozen

a college fund for the kids

starting a dream diary

the uncontrollable urge to lean out the car
    window and yell "Moo!" every time
    you pass a cow

taking an elevator friend to lunch

a shell collection and display case

handsome Greeks

putting on a bracelet without assistance

privacy

people who give more of themselves

conventional wisdom

the basic Vermont meal: a piece of
    Cheddar, a glass of cold milk,
    and a stack of common crackers

intramurals
the half-light of evening
regimental ties
mindful consuming
postcard views
saying, "Nice doggie"
someone who makes up
    for everything else
kick pleats
Hawaiian days and
    Las Vegas nights
lazing about
a rolltop desk
ergasiophobia, a fear of work
colorful markets
bagels and onion rolls
pepperoni pizza
cutting down on junk food
cheese pumpkins and sugar pumpkins
waking up Christmas morning and
    drinking hot eggnog
cushions of brushed denim
better results from order, form, and
    harmony
a hazy metropolitan skyline growing out
    of the horizon
an "I Miss You" note
a pot of steaming chili served with a
    dollop of sour cream and grated
    Cheddar in pottery bowls

the start of a good classical record
collection: Bach's *Brandenburg
Concertos*, Beethoven's *Symphony
No. 3*, Brahms's *Symphony No. 1*,
Chopin's *Piano Concerto No. 2*,
Debussy's *La Mer*, Handel's *Water
Music Suite*, Mozart's *Symphony
No. 40*, Stravinsky's *The Rite of
Spring*, Tchaikovsky's *Symphony
No. 6*, and Vivaldi's *Four Seasons*

boxer shorts and jockey shorts and briefs

notes for a book idea on a cocktail napkin

heading north

living in the place you love

Cajun music and Texas fiddle

antique crock-eye marbles

learning to say no

Christmas cookie cutters

new uses for old toothbrushes

nights of clanging bell buoys

winning a prize

sailing a dinghy

stock exchanges

a healthy economy

the sport of geocaching, a GPS-based
scavenger hunt

"And now for something completely
different." (Monty Python)

a chance to detox

the green shoots of new plants

the seat on the school bus directly over
    the rear wheel
"You turkey!"
breakers of the fast
a blissful hour of yoga in a great open
    space
folding chairs
air castles
celebrating this present moment
the herb butter-and-eggs
rain rattling the roof and banging at the
    window
frolicking
ski and snowboard wax
Sunday night family-room suppers
red licorice
trees noisy with songbirds
cookbooks with very readable type
a pretty table for a holiday meal
stew in a pottery pot
Home Box Office (HBO)
Grey Poupon mustard
refreshments
press boxes
describing what it's like to win a race
boutique candy stores
dwarf iris
big hair
children just learning to talk
hypnogogic jerks

electrifying colors
red rubber boots for walking through
the streets and woods after the rain
or snow and hearing the wonderful
sound your footsteps make
bone china
a purse that garners compliments
"I Can't Give You Anything but Love,
Baby" (song)
man walking on the moon (1969)
earning several doctorates
herbal hot pads
cake mix
unfringed jeans
food that means love
wolves' and dogs' pups
cleaning the whole house
pausing as you eat, by putting down your
utensils between bites
a birdwatcher's path
bar towels for polishing glassware
painting drawers different colors
listening to music so beautiful that it
makes you cry
roller-skating on the sidewalk
being more open, less helpless
bringing a bowl of berries to bed
the Earth's axis
woolen mills
old Marx Brothers movies

insulated bottles full of cider spiced with
    hot cinnamon
silk stockings
not having any cavities
spending time in the baby's nursery after
    everyone is sleeping
just being outside all day, doing nothing
doggie sighs
sharing clothes
scalloped coastlines
a veranda with picnic tables and
    expansive windows enabling diners
    to enjoy the wooded scenery
streetcars
your sketchbook as the ultimate souvenir
keeping the same babysitter for years
a snail's pace
the TV show you would most like to be on
a spackling spatula
Christmas cards from the Metropolitan
    Museum of Art
a tan people notice
the hotel notepad
taking baths
umbrellas and wet streets
horseback trips
talking to Siri, but wondering why she
    does not know anything
not being intimidated by the selection
    at a fancy cheese shop

a bus ticket to go across the country
a piece of jewelry you plan to buy
    someday
hearty borscht
when you and your friend say the same
    thing at the same time
hitching one's wagon to a star
ensuring success by counting on one in
    four things going wrong
scale models
uplights in bare winter trees
cow tails taking batting practice
wearing perfume when you're alone
    reading
church pews
University of Tampa and University of
    Hawaii
anticipating a challenging school course
roads winding through orchards
postprandial drinks
riding a train across America
incubating a creative project
when the meeting ends early
raiding the refrigerator
picking music for a slideshow
stuffed-crust pizza
a can of newer-colored tennis balls
what you like about your town
bowling alley employees
ethnography

lazy inner-tube floats on a looping river
an old pickup truck with the tailgate
down, a willow basket chock-full of
sandwiches, salads, and cheese, a jar
of pickles, a crock of honey, a loaf of
bread just baked that morning, a red-
and-white checkered tablecloth, and
sunshine pouring down through the
overhanging branches of a grand old
oak tree
changing your handwriting
tea towels
butterscotch sundaes and Pepsi together,
tasting like banana baby food
fern fossils
As the World Turns (soap opera)
"Not my circus. Not my monkeys." (Polish
expression)
"Well begun is half done."
watching the winning touchdown
getting catalogs in the mail
Beverly Shores, Indiana
the ecstatic experience
clodhoppers
driving as you wish your kids would
flowers thriving on love and friendly
words
places heavy with history
the *Ghostbusters* movies
Napa Valley Wine Train, California

coin jukeboxes

tent dresses

a supermarket cart left on a deserted beach

paved roads

peaked white umbrellas, linened tables, and a gurgling fountain

all the trappings of baking: large bowl of eggs, blender, box of oats, brush for melted butter, recipe books, tempting flavorings

air so crisp and clear, it draws you outdoors

barbecued beans

a boy and a boat in a bathtub

working better in dull weather

servicemen returning from abroad

a room with a view

playing hooky when it snows: making a snowman, going sledding, sticking out your tongue and catching snowflakes

Swiss cheese

a roll-arm sofa

inspiring work space

lemon ice cream and cake

earrings for every outfit

KP duty

a paddle ball in the Christmas stocking

spending a night on the water in a sailboat

the rambunctiousness of boys

little girls with their teddy bears
letting go of expectations
sun tea
allowing extra time
footsteps in the snow becoming laced
    traceries of purple shadows
root cellars
keyless entry systems
class-year numbers on sweaters or jackets
award frames
setting up an office
camp beds
interviewing a couple who have been
    married for 50 years
tumbling children on the beach
life, a stately march to sweet but unheard
    music
playing dumb
the 360-voice Mormon Tabernacle Choir
shower benches
things that look juicy
egg coddlers
being tickled
frat parties
going public
yummy reading
watching thoughts like a tennis player
    watches the ball
steering wheels
becoming a licensed pilot

making believe you're somewhere else,
    in a different era or role
pointelle knit
writing a screenplay
drawing on a graphics tablet
picking the fastest lane
hightailing it
pocket and sliding doors
the gearshift on a recliner
studying the lists of the Buddha
listening to kids' logic
grandma hair
big rigs
fox cubs wrestling in wild strawberries
being lost in a sea of relatives
doing things by the book
house-sitting
when you stop thinking about whatever
    is bugging you
different sizes of Santa Clauses
shunpiking
a group of friends in trick-or-treat
    costumes
a cold Arizona morning of cerulean skies
    and the medicinal smell of sage
open house at an elementary school
the stone pier of an old railroad bridge
the Earth moving about 18.5 miles per
    second in its orbit around the Sun
reveling in a lack of structure

facing the truth
the pause before the first applause
bicycling around an island
souped-up cars
the stroke of luck involved in sometimes
    not getting what you want
the snappy bustle of pelicans and donkeys
warmed bread
appreciating the good fortune of loved
    ones
lots of little balls of different flavored
    sherbet, icy cold and rousing
a tide chart at the local bait-and-tackle
    shop
string beans
old-fashioned English steak-and-onion pie
the metal clicker at the top of a ballpoint
    pen
thinking you lost your key card, then
    finding it
watching old movies with old friends
stopping an ant march into the house
things best done alone: poetry,
    performing, exercising, wallowing
quaking green aspen trees
loosening-up motions with the wrist
    before writing
zippered purses
when someone finally takes down their
    dead Christmas wreath in February

outdoor cafés on Chicago's Rush Street
and New York City's Columbus Avenue
getting back to the time when you
couldn't think of anything but each
other
fresh pleasure at being outside
ghost stories and marshmallows by a fire
hockey teams that use finesse rather than
brawn
smoked hams hanging on warped barn
rafters
talking heart to heart
a unifying principle
beards without mustaches still being
better than beards with mustaches
children poking sleepy heads out of dewy
tents
healing arts
beach huts
intelligent life on the planet Earth
alternating two exercise activities such as
yoga and walking
when salespeople admire the picture of
your mate or child in your wallet
stained glass
an old sled
plant descriptions on sticks
starting a show
turning things upside down to draw them
getting a passport

skinny Christmas trees
chalet-type motel units with their own
    balconies and view of the mountains
sun-reflector blankets
gallon cans of caramel
tossed salad
downspouts after a rain
tandem snow-shoveling projects
prom-goers working on their tans
dancing school: learning the fox-trot,
    waltz, cha-cha, rumba, merengue,
    eggbeater, and frug
the reassurance of being petted a little,
    praised a little, appreciated a little
notabilia, things worthy of note
touches of gold
a dream trip to Antarctica
feeding your mind
a Vermonter
meat carved at your table
long-stemmed glasses
al fresco, out of doors
weird dreams that make no sense
the original Girl Scout cookies
the kitchen of a famous restaurant
being an "anti-plastic" person
narrowly avoiding an animal that hesitates
    in the middle of the road
teaching assistants and fellows
Pokémon characters

airport suitcase tags

logos, graphics, whimsy, stenciling,
    trompe l'oeil, pen-and-ink renderings,
    painted primitives, and illustration

insulated food totes

the warm feeling of waking up on a cold
    morning and discovering you have
    another 20 minutes to sleep

Humphrey Bogart movies

candleshine

peppermint sticks

playing kissy-face

those who make us better people

the interests you pursue

a hometown of three houses and a cow

needlework stimulating deep thought

sequoia containing all five vowels

cathedral ceilings

printing a massive 3 x 4-foot photo
    (engineering print) at Staples

the pride we take in what we have
    contributed to our communities

a walk downtown

Nora Ephron, author

pinecones opening early

the cheerful feeling you have when
    nothing is troubling you

a rising middle moon

a delayed reaction to a situation or joke

Italian salad dressing

the traffic jam breaking up after a mile
Easter egg hunts
five-way Cincinnati chili
an orchard that supplies large plastic bags
and also labels which rows of trees
contain certain varieties
toga-ed Romans
life beginning at 40
a favor returned
seeing a grown man cry
jewelry pliers
sheet pizza and root beer
baseball coach signals
pastry carts
a soft summer's night
drawing a straight line freehand
North Dakota: durum and spring wheat,
wild birds, International Peace
Garden, churchgoers
a fireplace visible in two rooms
morning music
the magic of Adobe Photoshop
fruit trees in glorious clouds of red, white,
and pink
two-by-fours
soceraphobia (fear of in-laws)
making love on a secluded beach
garage-cleaning sessions
painters' hats
unsubscribing from junk email

pinking shears

monkeypod wood

all the days of your life when you have
     been healthy

letting bluffs be bluffs

alpine breezes

s'mores: chocolate and marshmallows
     melted between graham crackers

your default Web browser

the oxeye daisy

feeling empowered

bouquets of silk flowers all over the house

Idaho, the last of the 48 states to be
     explored

visiting the zoo in winter

a flashlight beam in the darkness

European soccer

fortune cookie: All your hard work will
     soon pay off.

"On a Clear Day," sung by Barbra Streisand

ratatouille

where the conversation gets good

"Finish each day and be done with it. You
     have done what you could. Some
     blunders and absurdities no doubt
     crept in; forget them as soon as you
     can. Tomorrow is a new day. You shall
     begin it serenely and with too high a
     spirit to be encumbered with your old
     nonsense." (Ralph Waldo Emerson)

liking the people you work with
books you've underlined
extra-large sizes, like 1X and 2X
chili in green peppers
a new millennium
spot checks
a five-year-old playing with Scotch tape
winter wheat
defrosting in a microwave
unsalted butter
astronauts
five o'clock shadow
eating candy bars at room temperature
blue corn chips in a turquoise bowl
healthy gums
feeling witty, confident, devastatingly sexy
throwing a coin in a well or fountain and
    making a wish
lip pencils, eye crayons
visiting Paris as a teenager
cream cheese frosting
corn butterers
"To err is human, to forgive is divine—
    but to forget is altogether humane."
Greenwich, Connecticut: "The Gateway to
    New England"
savoring a lake by canoe
cleaning out your wallet, makeup case,
    and purse
knowing how to get the most out of life

fried chicken with hushpuppies

bubbling cool springs

a miniature greenhouse for plants during frost season

deer staying in the woods

coleslaw dressing

a winter breakfast: steaming bowls of oatmeal topped with raisins or sliced bananas

stealing a few minutes to watch the clouds drift by your window and the leaves wafting in the breeze

buying enough candy for all the trick-or-treaters

the Bay of Fundy, with the highest tides in the world

doing a double take

nibbles

opening clams

nail glazes

pink peonies

beveling the edge of a mirror to add prisms of light

a spectacular ride over the swirling rapids of the Colorado River

platform-deck rockers

retiring with lots to do

pipe cleaners

knowing some self-defense techniques

pulling in the driveway after vacation

pinstripes

the hand movements of the hula

marina eateries

secret mazes

Reuben sandwiches and pickles

James Bond movies

being swept away by sheer delight

doing three or four crossword puzzles
until 3 a.m.

a pumpkin pie, light and pungent

bigheartedness

eating Chinese food from the takeout
containers

theater parties

exultant phone calls

a post office pen that writes

towels that absorb well

remembering a birthday

cheese, the oldest of manmade foods

a hippo having its teeth cleaned

seeing the thinnest sliver of the new moon
hanging in the sky at dusk

butter of the peanut

at a ball game, the smell of hot dogs and
ice cream and peanuts, the view of
the bleachers and the flags flying
overhead

a signing bonus

in summer, bayberry and eelgrass brushed
with sun

Coca-Cola commercials
getting sunkissed on lunch hour
throbbing downtowns
cricket matches
Ping-Pong
authoring or editing a Wikipedia article
foodie-traveler hot spots
taking your coffee on a walk
a cut that heals quickly
when you think you are out of candy but
then find one more left in the package
running a retail store
bacon-and-egg skillets
a corduroy couch
food for thought
sights that take your breath away
paint shirts
money-back guarantees
wind whipping the sand at the shore
of an ocean or a lake and piling it
into dunes
a weeklong stint at a farm school,
getting trained in organic gardening
and farming
crisp, batter-coated vegetables
owning your own barn
freshwater lakes
speaking your mind at a town meeting
riding on the crossbar of a bike late
at night

fragile, colorful butterflies fluttering
across the swaying grass
black pants
fireside conversations
the smell of freshly brewed coffee
puffins, kittiwakes, gannets, murres, and
sea parrots
swinging doors to the restaurant kitchen
diacritical marks
Davy Crockett, pioneer
grating some fresh Parmesan cheese
leaves in great golden drifts as crisp as
beaten gold foil
scavenger hunts
"Wheaties" as a nickname for an athlete
how life's daily events can entertain you
the original four flavors of Jell-O:
strawberry, raspberry, orange,
and lemon
a village street c. 1890, with old bricks,
wrought iron, bay windows, and
antique stained glass at the entrances
of stores
a smile from a stranger
Kissimmee, Florida
naming your baby
Rodgers and Hammerstein
interview shows
standing in the lake at sunset, holding
hands

having a scratch for every itch
setting a good example
pieces of life coming together like the
    scattered fragments of a jigsaw puzzle
turning over to even out your tan
how-come explanations
piano chords
crunch time
cocooning
daisies in the kitchen
peg and chalkboard desks
making your own trail mix
colorful workout clothes and stylish
    pajamas
miniature orange trees
people who travel in RVs
restored colonial homes
sugary lemonade
knowing your name in semaphore
casual, mobile, outdoor lifestyles
a shiny brass bucket full of pinecones that
    have been dipped in wax
butter-yellow sandstone
trying to figure it all out with a smile
dozens of acres of temples and statuary
    and steep-sided lakes concealed by
    centuries of vines
bylines on the front page
time to open the windows and let the
    street sounds mingle with your own

writing menus

kidding around with your child

sunlight filtering through panes of red,
blue, and yellow leaded glass

overlooking lighted cliffs of a bay

feeling good

isosceles trapezoids

lightning-white teeth

Greek vs. Italian pizza

a barometer telling tomorrow's weather

floor buffers

opposable thumbs

satellite navigation systems

buying the display model

microwave popcorn

HAL and Dave in *2001: A Space Odyssey*
(movie)

the art spirit

curtainless French doors

double ovens

a maraschino cherry and orange slice
stuck through a toothpick

an item without a price sticker

lattice-top pie crust

rich and fluffy unsugared whipped cream

a soothing array of musical instruments

clapping along

a pregnant goldfish

two people working together on making
a salad

natural beauty, history, botany, geology,
and sea life

stretching out on the carpet with games
and puzzles

when you see all the street lamps
turning on

the changing bits of colored glass in
a kaleidoscope

Cumberland Gap and Daniel Boone
country

backpack purses

getting only slightly sunburned on
a sailboat

paper logs

playing penny-ante poker

cinnamon-scented yams

people who work as hard as you do

inglenook, a corner by a fireplace,
the chimney corner

glacial lakes

tame animals: burro, camel, cat, cow,
dog, donkey, dromedary, goat,
horse, ox, pig, reindeer, yak

pan-roasted potatoes

guessing the pumpkin's weight and
getting it free

each inch of a garden revealing some
new life

ontology in information science

waterproof mittens

immediate materialization of the cat when
the food is brought out

rolling the package of bacon before
opening

Teva and Keen shoes

taking a walk downtown on Saturday
night to buy the Sunday *New York
Times*

fancy hankies

lichens arranged on a piece of wood

sweet dreams at the end of a journey
home

always accepting an outstretched hand

ribald humor

unusual toilet seats

toasted marshmallows, black outside,
squishy inside

sea otters

rereading old letters, magazines, and
books

being inside a tent in the woods

farewell kisses

the sky fading to a burning orange, the
moon popping out, and eventually the
thin crack of light under your door
flickering to black

Jell-O cakes

long Edwardian jackets

wondering what it would be like to be rich
and taken care of

a popcorn cart
treasures within a windowpane
billing and cooing
letting go of the gas pump perfectly
    so you end on a round number
a major drop in humidity
counting down NASA-style
building a fire pit
rock climbing instead of social climbing
putting Scrabble tiles in a jar and then
    dumping out 10 tiles and making a
    word to jump-start an idea
people-watching from a park bench
wraparound sunglasses
things that fortify the spirit
decorating paper plates
down quilts
late fall, when men move indoors like
    bears to doze before the TV
the look on someone's face when he
    or she realizes they are on the big
    screen at the game
Bugs Bunny
having a baby's sneakers bronzed
tins of homemade Christmas cookies
Kyle Rote, football player
Keir Dullea, actor
when mellow days turn into
    brisk evenings
jellybeans in an Easter basket

tricolored gold stackable rings
learning the best methods for doing things
in the kitchen
spending a lunch hour in a beautifully
planted, air-conditioned atrium
the Gregorian calendar
mushy talk
what you deem indispensable
blueberry soup
"mix well" as life's motto
rich, smooth cheesecake
evergreens, wearing winter's ermine
gracefully
jars to collect things in
leafing through boxes of unsorted
photographs
looking toward tomorrow
kitchen chores
listening to someone excitedly tell a story
locating the fountain of youth
Donald Duck
vintage cabs
eating the sugar left in the bottom of the
coffee cup
wandering into an antique furniture store
the song of someone in the shower
little luxuries
the haven you escape to for hours: sitting
curled there, dreaming, reading,
building yourself a life, a world

ski jumping

the roar of a crowd

videoconference calls

Steamboat Willie, starring Mickey Mouse
in 1928

a bacon press

the polar seas

happiness being the atmosphere in which
all good affections grow

the almost subliminal awareness of a
gestating idea

layers of clouds stacked in the sky

playing the percentages

restorative yoga

presidential nominations and
inaugurations

the smell of popcorn and hot roasted
peanuts

being off the beaten track

relaxed-fit and comfort-waist jeans

the art of conversation

trying a new sleeping schedule

the world's deepest, darkest places,
inhabited by some of the strangest-
looking animals on the planet

small processes, interactions, and
relations changing by the nanosecond

Cartoon Network marathons

Windsor ties

weird biology teachers

busy times

a snowdrift curled in the shape of the
storm's breath

whittling life down to 100 still-to-be-read
books, a few pairs of jeans, some
cotton shirts, and socks

sunsets/starry nights/full moons

sleeping with a jacket over you

knees quivering when your lover walks in

the ivy walls of Wrigley Field

a sleepy fishing village

being sent home from work early

yellow beach bicycles

an adventure such as a hike, ice-skating,
or a football game

a handy stool for out-of-reach cabinets

sweet-and-sour carrots

being comfortable with silence

varsity letter jackets

soufflé-light pashmina

other people's doodles

soda water

respectfully yours

country house visiting

playing dodgeball with a Nerf ball

Ray Charles, musician

two for the price of one

Saturday lunch for leaf-rakers

dreaming of dancing at the royal ball and
midnight never comes

the middle of a lake
broad-leaved evergreens
clearing the underbrush
remaining calm as if nothing
    happened
sliced bread
frolicking in a pile of leaves
the ketchup patch on a plate
drying gourds
hands-free-everything public bathrooms
nervy people
trees caught napping
meeting someone special at the customs
    gate
afternoon air that dares you to breathe it
bamboo stilt houses
brushstrokes in artists' pastels
the Montauk Point lighthouse
strangers you see so regularly that you
    feel they're almost friends
taffy-pulling contests
ropes slapping against a flagpole
beacon lights
a cream-colored wool tennis pullover with
    navy and maroon stripes
the thought that one door closes and
    another one opens
cantilevered and double-hung staircases
setting wise priorities
nontoxic paint

pausing in the damp marsh of a bogland
among the marsh marigolds
obsidian
leaves that are still, not whispering
freewheeling characters
seedless black raspberry preserves
only one macaroni salad at the potluck
seeing all your friends again on the first
day of school
long hair
Boy Scouts making a fire
waylaying your latest crush on the
footbridge
the millions of What if? questions
dinner with laughter
a slice of lemon that fits perfectly in the
top of a glass of Perrier
Hear! Hear!
seeing a drawing in relation to the
drawing paper, the lightness or
darkness of each line, the crispness
or fuzziness of each mark
a special moment in time
autosuggestion
a Subway sandwich run
studying a student pilot's manual
a jazz brunch
putting things back where they were
found
waves and sea spray through a sea arch

heavy-duty shelving

letters from close friends in far places

romantic beds

a cold Arctic wind ripping red and gold leaves from the trees

unscarred snow

when a sibling lifts your spirits

bucolic scenery

eating what you like and letting the food fight it out inside

old travel and movie posters

learning about soil types and grape varieties

bread rising

muffins bought at a bakery while biking through Martha's Vineyard

basement family rooms

crossover basketball dribbling

heavenly sights like dreams created

being camera-shy

special commemorative magazines

sunny yellow napkins

"I scream, you scream, we all scream for ice cream."

looking at everything and everybody around you as though you're seeing them for the first time

peeking out from under sunglasses

living each day for itself

squeezing limes

the tide edging homeward once more
tissue paper
updating your computer's operating
    system without any big problems
buying Christmas decorations early
lowering your monthly bills
a group of long-stemmed goblets filled
    with fresh flowers
an old-fashioned wooden trencher (plate)
Pallas's cats in a Himalayan pass
Huck and Jim
potluck recipes
the feel of a rug under bare feet
French toast, butter, and powdered sugar
taking a walk when the world is too much
the inability to stop spelling the word
    banana once you've started
sending an April Fools' telegram
recreation department meetings
steaming cups of Darjeeling or Earl Grey
painting your own greeting cards for
    special people
babbling brooks
an inaudible slurp while eating spaghetti
planning a pond
klieg lights
no-turning-back situations
business sense
sweet-smelling pine on the fire
working at/from home

balls of real butter
the first run of a play
Montego Bay, Jamaica
putting new fleece inserts in your slippers
sportswriting
a clever Google Doodle for the day
alacrity—cheerful willingness, liveliness
scanning a star-filled sky on a still winter
    night
the sandpapering action of moraines and
    glaciers
brushing the dew from sneakers
looking at each tabletop as a still life
classy nightclubs
memory lane
keeping an "I love you" note in your desk
Earth shoes
the original Podunk, the area between
    Hartford and Windsor, Connecticut
eating a ripe peach and letting the juice
    trickle down your chin
entertaining, if you like to
the art of candymaking
that week each month when most
    monthly magazines hit the stands
telecommuters
a sun-toasted colonnade
crab cakes with remoulade sauce
impala bucks
the Twister game

Meet the Press (TV show)

pomanders grouped with pinecones,
    mandarin oranges, and gourds

jewelry repaired while you wait

Venus, both the closest planet to Earth
    and the planet closest in size to Earth

apartments

sound collage

the thrush singing at twilight and the
    nightingale by moonlight

the Golden Rule

growing onions

the first hours of sunlight: time to twinkle
    and strike sparks from frosty twigs
    and icy ponds, time to pencil long
    shadows on every tree-lined meadow

savoring an achievement

fair use

a mission-driven discipline

the perfect piece of chocolate cake

game birds

Jack Kornfield, Buddhist teacher

April chills

moonbeams on the water, like fairies
    spawned from light

the orange balls on power lines

having the time to reread *Little Women*
    and *Psycho-Cybernetics*

writing in the sand

ancient alphabets

the third log for making the fireplace light
when physical fitness was related only to
    gym class and President Kennedy
silos, like giant thermoses on the
    dairyland table
the intimacy of humor
investing your money
making peace
British English
boroughs of the City of New York
speedwriting
parallel and crisscross styles of lacing
    sneakers
the light inside the refrigerator
a thoughtful thought
not worrying about what's going to
    happen
the Milky Way
unique comments in a guest register for
    an event
the rising of the sun on a misty morning
the acoustic version
mirrored objects
archaeology at Monticello
a milkshake served on a glass plate with
    doily, vanilla cookie, straw, spoon,
    and metal container of more
circuit breakers
fish fillets
brand-new automobile tires

Norman Rockwell art
giving yourself credit
zills, finger cymbals used by belly dancers
overhead compartments on airplanes
Burger King and Wendy's Fun Meals
the 275 waterfalls of Iguacú Falls on the
    border of Argentina and Brazil
swallowing your pride
lunch boxes
selling all your junk on eBay and making
    a profit
when push-button telephones were new
housecleaning your mental crannies
taking in a stray puppy
a scented herb pressed into a book
afternoon tea in London
making it halfway through something
reading the newspaper
prize finds
finger paintings
a childhood platform swing
connecting with someone new
seeing old people holding hands
disco dancing
covered butter dishes
toast with maple cream
camp-style meals
bodies of water that collect on upturned
    mugs in the dishwasher
straight-from-the-dyepot blue Bahamian sky

a ripe apricot
a potbellied-stove kind of day
cutting through a park
thinking counterintuitively
a loud-color pair of pants
seeing a preview version
chilled orange or tomato juice
moonshiners' copper stills
laughing as you remember good times
    together
revelers in satin and taffeta
foot traffic
a filled refrigerator
doing something nice for someone
    without letting on that you did it
funny get-well cards
refreshing philosophy and original wisdom
the cheery noise of bubbling pancake
    batter
petri dishes
20-ton Olmec heads
mushroom farms
pulling all bedcovers as close as possible
    to keep away ghosts, goblins, and
    burglars
favorite aunts
a first name that goes well with a last
    name
zarf, a holder for a handleless coffee cup
a trip to the library

rain for the yard

the person at theaters who tears tickets

a tan in April

a carousel with hand-carved animals and
2,000 lightbulbs

apple-pie order

the ubiquity of poinsettias

circular lakes

the phenomenon of dust

basic recipes

your ship coming in

a pitcher of water with sliced lemon in the
refrigerator

team pictures

cracks in the sidewalk

The New York Times Book Review

toboggan slides

vine fruits

candy tins

a 10-gallon jug of fruit salad

mood rings

vision checks

doing the common things in life in an
uncommon way

ski knickers

ungodly hours

growing as our love grows

blue-glazed stoneware canisters, corked
and numbered *un* to *cinq* in a French
country kitchen

turning an -ophobe into an -ophile

back soothers

spending an hour in a casino and then
    vamoosing

ocean scallops sautéed in a very delicate
    curried drawn butter

the smell of damp, fresh-cut lumber

diminutive forms of words

the gift of attentive silence

Anne Frank's *The Diary of a Young Girl*

melting the ice

trying every ride at the carnival

the adaptive unconscious

folding the newspaper into quarters to do
    the crossword

the nod when you are cycling and
    someone goes past and it's like,
    "Hey, let's be friends for a second!"

kittens spanking sunbeams

the craziest person in your life

water fountains

a rectangular pizza

the alphabet by code: Alpha, Bravo,
    Charlie, Delta, Echo, Foxtrot, Golf,
    Hotel, India, Juliet, Kilo, Lima, Mike,
    November, Oscar, Papa, Quebec,
    Romeo, Sierra, Tango, Uniform,
    Victor, Whiskey, X-Ray, Yankee, Zulu

forecasting the weather

a well-stocked supermarket

coffee served with a
   pitcher of thick cream
dishes of beach glass
the Nixon transcripts
hardworking waiters
forever-green dieffenbachia plants
"Love lets the other be, but with affection
   and concern." (R.D. Laing)
Mr. Fixit
singing to your favorite music
ice carving
the giving of gifts
sunlight creating a dappled pattern
   through the trees
when things are hunky-dory or
   okey-dokey
barbecued chicken, mashed potatoes,
   and corn
sporty, casual, exciting, fresh, up, jaunty
   feelings
the children's latest school crafts projects
a crazy theory that turns out to be correct
a notebook for moving
treasuring the "ride"
the gentle mood of a lovely spring
   remembered
chain letters
a solo canoe or kayak trip
passing a course in art history
"America the Beautiful" (song)

blazing a trail

daring to be eccentric

Troy and Heinrich Schliemann's finds

reflecting at the beach

questions designed to provide revealing
insights into our psyches

visiting the grocery store, church, and
library in your hometown

massive quartz veins in rocks

world globes

neon hypercolor shirts

leaving the mistletoe up all year

a wall-hung dispenser for plastic wrap,
foil, and paper towels

a rabbit's foot

the art of bonsai and using bonsai scissors

old report cards

tear-stained pillows reminding you that
times always get better

Marshall Field's store, Chicago

drying racks for clothes

a child's sandbox

twilight victory parties

Williamsburg, Virginia

long-distance calls

taking a maraschino cherry from the bar
while paying the tab

the Gulf Stream

clean kids' sneakers

leftover flower children

made-on-the-farm taste
fishing boats blanketing a beach
electromagnetic energy
official scorekeepers
tender-textured yellow muffins
dragging your heels a bit
being inventive in placing groceries
    in a tiny sports car
making friends with a dog
a bike helmet as hard as the carapace
    of a turtle
lighted makeup mirrors
the blatant lies and illogic that mothers
    use to discourage "dangerous"
    activity among children
visiting an uninhabited island
miniature bowling games in
    bowling alleys
ice-cream pops, Eskimo pies,
    Good Humor
great cats named Hoops and Hooper
getting B's in a math course like geometry
riding bikes in school parking lots
slalom racing
the northern wilderness
a tropical fish tank
something free for the asking
the difference between annuals and
    perennials
mustard seed

gazpacho in the summer

quiet

taking something apart and discovering
just how many parts it takes to make
the whole—and that the whole is
much more than the sum of the parts

meandering

when everyone had address books

a binge day

proposing a special project

watching someone take a nap

scoop scales

tartan blankets

dog walking

travel journals

18th-century merchant princes' homes

a covered woodpile

melt-in-your-mouth food

when our children exceed our own
achievements

that feeling when you can't wait to tell
someone something

the confidence of a smooth operator

a farmer's tan in the spring

the next tick of the clock

books that matter to you

provolone cheese

when there's a thick gray rim of thawing
ice lining the streets

watching river barges negotiate a lock

collared sweatshirts
aquarium light
formal gardens
warming up a pen to get it to start writing
sailing out of the clouds
grilled cheese and fries
mixed vegetables in onion sauce
baskets of eggs
maple, butternut, apple, and locust trees
the Hokey-Pokey
crab soccer and getting your hands filthy
    playing it
inviting guests
musty old books
rings exchanged at a wedding
the force of habit
what gives you comfort right now
cats darting through alleyways
beach and weekend houses
wax vampire teeth
a trunk full of patchwork pieces
white leather
Hawaiian pizza's pineapple and ham
secret passages
live music drifting from a dockside pub
movies with wagon trains
Chia Pets
cat doors or flaps
abundance
sponge or color-blot paintings

making time to meditate
looking at dish patterns
the Memphis Belle
wild-cherry orchards
sleeping naked between crisp sheets
picnic areas with campfire circles
St. Mark's Square in Venice
on Christmas Eve, a stocking on each
    guest's chair filled with funny and
    special gifts pertaining to each one's
    interests
fish tank bubbles
a passenger-seat dog
soft lagoons by moonlight
a private collection of pleasures
stapling a finished essay together
the heightened awareness of the sheer joy
    of nature, the stillness, the changing
    patterns of light and shade, the small
    sounds of honeybees, the gentle
    cooing of doves
sun porches
pearl earrings
being frugal
spending a great deal of time walking the
    boards of your porch
dicing onions
the start of softball season
The Linnaeus Garden in Uppsala
responsibly marking your trail

smoke curling out of 200-year-old
   chimneys
a successful kid's birthday party
exotic Chinese birds hand-painted on
   cotton
ideas about purse design
training wheels
the journey of a lost dollar
willows that look like great honey-colored
   fountains
a spectacular massage
rote memory
a bookcase end table
20 shades of green in a tree
baseball hats
pewter casting
enjoying the aroma before
   your first sip
snowbound towns
beach umbrellas
flour sifters
egg cartons
that irresistible, clean-baby smell
an autumn centerpiece
mental files
mailing five sheets of paper with one
   stamp
a sprig of sea hollyhock
uses for dishwashing detergent
whipped cupcake icing

falling crazily, I'd-kill-or-be-killed-for-that-
	person in love
interesting reproductions
buying a good dictionary
piecrusts made with lard
artistic license
the great amphitheater at Epidaurus,
	Greece
fruitcake tins
the first few seconds of warmth from a
	blazing fire
a simple holiday party
Shetland sweaters in ice blue, sawdust,
	Oxford gray, hunter green
bending over backward
the yelp of a puppy
French francs
collecting kindling with a child on a crisp
	autumn afternoon
a tripod for family photos
Mercedes taxicabs and limousines
the rich, earthy smell of a garden,
	actinomycetes at work
spring breaks on Martha's Vineyard
a surprise burst of joy
early rays of sun peeking through wispy
	clouds
the soft feel of cotton sheets
pink butcher's paper
keeping a stash of stocking stuffers

the small rubbery pads on the bottom of
a cat or dog's paws

taking a long walk someplace quiet and
making up lyrics to songs

swimming in a country club pool

pita bread with very thin roast beef and
Greek salad

washing out bathing suits

devouring a book in one sitting

albino watermelon seeds

flowers basking

holding hands under a table

where the good times are

counting your blessings

library exploration

fines herbes

Arby's, Baskin-Robbins, Burger King,
Carvel, KFC, Dairy Queen, Dunkin'
Donuts, McDonald's, Taco Bell,
Wendy's, White Castle

potato latkes

wormholes, hypothetical tunnels in
space-time

parcel post and media mail

a plan of action

ad absurdum and ad nauseam

the go-ahead to write a book

boiled egg, orange juice, toast, jam, huge
strawberries, 18th-century hot-milk
jug, pot of coffee

remembering when all soda came in
     bottles and had sugar in it
the first time a new friend calls you
     by your nickname
making faces at monkeys in the zoo
nipping something in the bud
vocal percussion in an a cappella chorus
the hundred voices of a January wind
an "idea person" at your disposal
winks
Neuschwanstein Castle in Germany
the Candyland game
fried green tomatoes with bacon and
     cheese
the tools that help you get your job
     done—computer mouse, coffee,
     dictionary, copier, brain, thesaurus,
     tape, Moleskines, pens, cat
letting someone make you laugh
kitchen timers
art: the wine of life
hiring a housekeeper
"the green stuff"
cat footprints on a car window
good things coming your way
seeing an apple fall from a tree
cable-knit socks
Maine clams
a flawless sea
collegiate functions

tulips pushing through rain-soaked soil

a moss terrarium

exotic fresh fruits served cosseted in
    bowls of vanilla cream

a wedge of iceberg lettuce with bacon,
    cherry tomato, and Roquefort

the best farmhouse butter

the gracious laugh or smile

being clear-eyed

blankets of white coating sidewalks like
    icing

pulling out a weed and its roots

a porch swing cradling a puddle of cat

shirt jackets

windowsill planters

showing initiative

a really good workout at home

dancin' in the moonlight

a coming-out-of-hibernation hike

the momentary thrill of sitting on a washing
    machine as it goes into spin cycle

glisteny stuff

cotton-velour terry wrap robes

being recognized for doing your own thing
    and respected for it

plenty of kitchen shelves

a photo collage

making an ice-cream pie

shoeless Saturdays

wood lathe art

sinking a turnaround jumper

long, fat yellow ears of sweet corn

diving right in

the person who studies the menu but
orders the same thing every time

sound resonating

in-a-nutshell reports
that things are replaceable

someone who puts his or her arm
around you

post offices

large sandwiches alternately called
heroes, wedges, submarines, hoagies,
grinders, or poorboys

self-cleaning pets

animals at their watering troughs

walking to work

sketching in a field

birth certificates

ivy-leaved toadflax stretching to a bank of
wild strawberries

over-the-sink cutting boards

nonstop cool

clover waking and rising in the morning in
a slow, unfaltering stretch

riding a steam train around the park
periphery

the janitor gently sweeping the school

setting up the dining room table for arts
and crafts

leaves becoming a restless golden drift, a
     wine-red flurry in the wind
popcorn-and-tears movies
a waiter who is concentrating
everything sticking its head out in spring
cutting your TV viewing in half
grandmas: moms with lots of frosting
electric toothbrushes
foreign stamps
planning a camping trip
clean windows
rosy mornings
the discovery of sunken ships
panning a scene
new babies
party spreads
anniversaries remembered
     with flowers, gifts, or cards
running a booth at a fair
"American Pie" by Don McLean
Boris Badenov and Natasha Nogoodnik,
     archenemies of Rocky and Bullwinkle
choosing not to be tattooed
the little hole in the sink that lets water
     drain out instead of flowing over the
     side, called a porcelator
your usual chair
the multiverse
not minding the silences
a good ear doctor

buying all new pencils and pens
retracing Thoreau's three-day canoe trip
road daisies
wooden beads
northern lights
staying friends with those who are miles
    away
an old-fashioned soapstone griddle
afternoon pick-me-ups
"Auld Lang Syne" by Guy Lombardo
the sound of feet crunching through new
    snow or frozen leaves
having a green thumb
the reverberation of a school bell
nursing a drink
when the mountains are calling
typing something on a cell phone or tablet
    and not having to go back and correct
    most of the words
eating ice-cream sandwiches by first
    licking around the sides
people leaning on the counter, reading the
    newspaper
Crayolas plus imagination
organizing a sleigh ride
pearly whites
the satisfaction of fully exerting yourself
curled trees
an authentic, artistic, and aesthetic life
broiled corn on the cob

Blue Rhythm painting by Hans Hofmann
ordering a cord of wood
one of those icy-brittle mornings when
    sounds carry far
cookie cutters
elephant jokes
following a pony trail
cigar boxes
the huge ladders on fire trucks
Indian pudding served warm with a big
    scoop of vanilla ice cream
a plan to mend a quarrel between friends
starting where you are
robust parades
two million years, a geological eye blink
laugh lines
poolside tables
well-designed school lockers
a square dance
being remembered long after the holidays
    are forgotten
bristlecone pine, the oldest (acknowledged)
    living organism
great halftime bands
soft flour tortillas with chili, cheese, and
    lettuce
gently floodlit trees
cooking your first turkey
popover pans
cats named Hamburger and Cheeseburger

torrential downpours

sap buckets

self-sufficient hardy people

"Happy Birthday!" yelled as you enter
a crowded room

models' bags

church lofts

ripening fruit

a belief that caution often deserves to be
thrown to the wind

a 3-mile-long mini railroad

the phrase "Let a camel get his nose under
the tent and he'll come in."

Maine snowshoe furniture

being shipwrecked with your overnight
bag

tractor feet

tyke bikes

the crisp, secret rustle of a whispering
breeze in a cornfield

aviation windsocks

gulls swooping and scolding

having a mudroom

the rhythms of speech, the blend of deep
and shrill voices, the medley of laughs

Vogue magazine

wedding vows by the ocean

bacon slabs

hearing someone's heart beat

the best things said coming last

soda-pop bubbles

a place of golden canyons, apricot sands, terra-cotta mountains, and mauve shadows

staring at the figures on restroom doors to determine men's and women's

sudsy water

places to go antiquing

pottery made of different-colored clays for a marbled or mottled effect

how the brain binds data supplied by the senses and memory

butter streusel coffeecake

the Missing Link

Pictionary and Cranium games

pets under the blankets

a lakefront you visited as a child

knocking someone's socks off

putting clean clothes away

dangling upside down

typing into a search box

steak joint/rock-Muzak places

doing your job well

university dairy bars, especially in New England

the slow light of a late dawning

red-brown stoneware pots

Pennsylvania scrapples

when tulips and daffodils start appearing in grocery stores

Capoeira, a martial art combining
elements of music and dance
pulling up your collar
a group of teammates jumping together
houses built of butter-colored limestone
watching the snow from your office
colors of the 64-crayon box: carnation
pink, salmon, lavender, thistle, orchid,
periwinkle, blue-violet, violet, plum,
magenta, red, maroon, violet-red, red-
violet, mulberry, brick red, orange-
red, red-orange, melon, orange, burnt
orange, yellow-orange, apricot, peach,
maize, goldenrod, orange-yellow,
lemon yellow, yellow, yellow-green,
green-yellow, spring green, sea
green, green, olive green, pine green,
forest green, blue-green, green-blue,
turquoise blue, aquamarine, sky blue,
navy blue, cornflower blue, cadet
blue, midnight blue, blue, blue-
gray, violet-blue, raw sienna, sepia,
bittersweet, raw umber, brown, tan,
burnt sienna, mahogany, Indian red,
copper, silver, gold, gray, white, black
tiny balls of kid socks in a dresser drawer
bills of sale
stopwatches for track meets
a waterfall with submerged colored lights
that excited birthday-party feeling

a windsurfing regatta
being softly propped up in bed
beachside yoga
walking at the same speed as an
    elderly person so he or she
    does not feel rushed
7X, Coca-Cola's secret ingredient
laughing at yourself
secondhand books
wading through paperwork
cottage-fried potatoes
coffee for the commute
cranberry shrubs
rows of glass-fronted boutiques
gumdrop breaks
making a gutsy call
girl bands
the Hawaiian Islands
batter-fried zucchini and
    ranch dressing
the phone ringing on a rainy day
appreciating advantages
test tubes
a level playing field
sheltered nooks
chalk-white walls and floors of red tile
a ceremony about to begin
talkathons and walkathons
looking for an answer
a wicker food cover for outdoors

jigsaw puzzle setup: dumping out all the
    pieces on a card table, turning them
    all over, and propping up the picture
nourishment
a plane landing safely after a bumpy flight
the posting of the cafeteria's weekly menu
saying the word *thistle*
pharmacy floor lamps
thermal underwear to wear under your
    nightgown
fixing a rift in your family
your own energy as a letter of
    introduction
driving on a smooth road
sneaking off to the mountains in the
    middle of the week
having a sense of your own space
being kind to the child in you
needing a little love
opening a bottle of wine just for
    yourself and cooking a good
    dinner for one to go with it
the 100-meter dash
soaking in a scented tub
the undersides of furniture
the position of leaves on trees
being a graduate student
the Great Barrier Reef
smoke from the cookfire
the San Diego Zoo

windows close to the floor

monkey bars at the park

giving today all the love and intensity and
courage you can, traveling honestly
along life's path

a bibliophile's dream: a massive library of
his or her own

fog mists over violet moors

primitive and untouched things

the lonely sound of a train horn

the rewards of introspection

watching skaters on ponds

baskets made of woven strips of
construction paper, tied with ribbons
and filled with sugar cookies

full green vineyards

the hearth broom

the glow of streetlight scattered

dry-erase markers and white boards

"I love you" mouthed across a room

letting the story be told

tennis on clay courts

consciousness studies

someone laughing

a meeting where excitement builds
for an idea

striped ticking fabric

busy-day meals

puppy love

Philadelphia ready-to-eat cheesecake filling

redwood tables

Hamburger Helper

seeing Manhattan outside the train compartment window

marble occurring in a single belt extending from Stratford, Connecticut, through the Berkshires and western Vermont, to Lake Champlain

blowing straw wrappers across tables

creamy coleslaw

the little flaps or windows of an Advent calendar

a new yellow Volkswagen Beetle

little moments captured in photographs

Sedona, Arizona

rustic, weathered boards and planks

your favorite color palette

mini fireplace bursts

making sure you have your lucky charm

in-laws with "a life"

anything simple that you can do well and easily

experimental theater

a turtlet, a baby turtle

miles of dense virgin forest, laced with lakes and waterfalls

seeing a red fox traverse the backyard

pretending that you are a leaf drifting along a quiet, lazy stream on a sunny day

mother-of-pearl in an abalone shell

kosher pickles

cheese-stuffed green chili peppers dipped in egg batter and deep-fried, then topped with onions, sauce, and cheese

making a ship-in-a-bottle from a wine bottle, pieces of pine, thread, glue, pins, toothpicks, and ribbons for sails

a healing word or touch

throwing open your mind's shutters and letting the wind rush in— brainstorming, doodling, thinking, playing, daydreaming free-range

a perfect metaphor

sunshine coming through a window

using pokers to pick up paper

the Eastern seaboard

R-E-S-P-E-C-T

literacy

tweedy faculty types

tree-lined streets, fireflies, nighttime sounds, and aromas stirring up feelings of nostalgia

Dairy Queen Dilly Bars

the catch of the day

winning free tickets to an event

the vocabulary of sports announcers

gifts at graduation time

writing in the out-of-doors

oyster shucking

the calendar on soap operas that allows
one day's events to be stretched over
a three-week period

flower sellers arranging their wares in
the town square

nunchi, the subtle art and ability of
listening to and gauging others'
moods

bees filling the air with the buzz of
industry

learning how to drive a stick shift

the pep-rally atmosphere

a person with a fine work ethic

interjections

when unplugging the router for
30 seconds fixes the problem

getting out of a rut

the quick flash of deer startled by the
orchard's windfall

flying kites in the bold March sky

recognizing John Lennon's voice decades
later

remembering to do a task without having
to write it down

the hum of a freezer

a pinball-lit pizza emporium

the first maple leaf drifting down

those dear to you

a pig sleeping on its right side

short-order talk
Silicon Valley
seeing with new eyes
farmers and countrymen in the pub
sports banquets
a digital guitar tuner
pulling rank
free rein
the genetic code underlying life
waking up and being able to go back
    to sleep
fish and chips in a vinegary newsprint cone
the oath of office
taking the time to plump your dog's
    L.L. Bean doggy bed
gold rice-paper ceilings
leaving home, following your dreams, and
    returning enriched by the experience
breeze-swept rooms
minarets
hitting a tennis ball against the wall for
    practice
winding canals
library lights on the tops of bookshelves
open ocean, snug harbors, picturesque
    fishing boats, and gorgeous rocks
plant-sitting for a friend
salad pizza
homemade bread and real whipped butter
    for dinner

the racket of rolling garbage cans
bowling a strike in the last frame
chipmunks with their tails sticking
    straight up in the air
the argument that knowledge is never
    really acquired
needlepoint becoming habit-forming
tuna salad at a restaurant
churros from a warehouse store
a baby's vocabulary
candelabras entwined with garlands
    of holly
gentle head and shoulder rolls
the weird world of virtual reality
mint sherbet
quiet humaneness
Batman's enemies: Catwoman, the Joker,
    the Penguin, the Riddler
the plunk of a ball in a mitt
reading all night and sleeping all morning
relaxation and a chance to let down
a room that overlooks the high fields at
    the rear of an inn or resort
propagating bulbs
the sting of salt air
old-school waitresses
things that are better at night
wonton soup and California roll
the first drops of rain
freshly threshed wheat, oats, and barley

falling in love again

someone who leaves a light on for you

quid pro quo

vaulted rooms

a snorkel box (drive-up mailbox)

sitting outside in New England in early
February in 50°F weather

pearl onions

knowing to keep many of your thoughts
to yourself

old-fashioned hospitality

moving stuff around to make a room
look fresh

city squares

Great Britain

making something new

the 1962 Third Edition of *Roget's
Thesaurus*

one-room schoolhouses

a four-season porch

what you are willing to sacrifice to
become what you would like to be

first impressions

"As the archeology of our thought easily
shows, man is an invention of recent
date." (Michel Foucault)

finally getting off the ground

having a guesthouse

confiture, preserved or candied fruit

lovely sounding words

a toddler napping with his blankie
putting new mulch out in the spring
Ellery Queen mysteries
the priorities of college kids changing as
soon as college is over
the metal lunch box with a matching
thermos bottle
an original idea that demands your attention
an alarm clock that would tell you when
to wake up—and why
cake-and-lemonade parties
a computerized grocery list
a book wall
unique designs
vats of salad and cauldrons of soup
the crimson hues of October evenings
Audubon Society photographs
really great earplugs
a cocked hat
Harvard beets
being attracted to someone when you
least expect it
spending 15 percent of your workday
pursuing speculative new ideas
a bucket filled with little bunches of
flowers that perfectly combine all
of nature's colors
amino acids
settling down in a deep sofa and ordering
a cup of tea

extra-summery clothes

thumbprint art

an underground lake or river

cheesecake and espresso

being kind to a person who can do you
absolutely no good

a private end-of-the-road location

sports arenas

complimentary newspapers

communicating in a foreign country with
"yes," "no," "please," "thank you,"
"that," and numbers

the groan of ice on a lake when the
temperature has flirted with zero
all week

the nickname "Puddin' Face"

drinking hot water with lemon

mashed-potato sandwiches

get-away-from-it-all-and-relax times

measuring snow

dance school

when you are astonished

arguing a case before the Supreme Court

University of Notre Dame

when you are in a zone—literally—in a
sport you love, where time slows
down and you can hear absolutely
nothing

being a millionaire

je ne sais quoi

dressing your age

abundant wild grapevines

holding hands

being part of a research team

the witching hour

when the low, raking light of the sun picks
out the mountains and crater walls in
sharp definition

Ultimate Frisbee

the lowest zip code, 00501 (Holtzville,
New York), and the highest, 99950
(Ketchikan, Alaska)

a school of fish

floral-pattern furniture or pillows
enlivening the scholarly atmosphere
of a library

swallows returning

your own private slice of beach

lunching at a good restaurant in the city

sinecure, a position requiring little work
but with profitable returns

stick figure drawings

a power nap to increase your ability to
concentrate and learn

a black-and-white speckled spaghetti
cooker

natural language processing

polished stones

good evenings

zucchini fritters with lime mayo

age and beauty

short ski-lift lines

blinking and not missing something

the supreme beauty of mathematics

staying fresh

movie stories: temptation, rags to riches,
riddle, metamorphosis, rescue,
tragedy, love, monster force, revenge,
transformation, fish out of water,
maturation, pursuit, rivalry, underdog,
discovery, escape, journey and return,
comedy, quest, sacrifice, wretched
excess

running amok

dainty sandwiches with the crusts
trimmed off

Upwords and Derivation board games

caring for your paintbrushes

learning to like yourself better

Teflon frying pans in the back of the
cupboard from college days

fog burning off into a beautiful sunny day

the second cup of coffee

summer school dances

what a goodnight kiss can do for your
dreams

post-election parties

men who shave every day

anything that turns 100 and becomes an
official antique

a sunset with someone
house trailers
braking for rainbows
winning streaks
Barbie Doll weddings
paper lanterns
ham and Swiss cheese
phosphenes: the light you see when you
    rub your closed eyes
crazy socks peeking out
hash browns, paprika-spiced and salted
travel brochures for Greece
a small, attractive courtyard built around
    a gazebo
privately renewed wedding vows
spring peepers
pachysandra instead of grass
relaxing with a half hour of yoga
self-sticking stamps and labels
Memphis pork barbecue
shoveling without injuring yourself
going back to the drawing board
telling someone your dreams and
    fantasies
taxi medallions
esprit de corps
pecan pralines
using dried summer flowers in winter
    cards and letters
saving money regularly

reaching 70 years old
film studios
a canopied pontoon boat
Grade A eggs
a trellis of sweet peas
closing time
envelope sizes
a winding staircase
hooded and zippered sweaters
whistling a duet together
cuticle cream
memories sitting like lonely men on the
    park bench of the mind
Rock, Paper, Scissors
playground picnics
two Slinkies in love
sugar packets
driving to the beach with the windows
    wide open and music blaring
eating the cookie batter before it makes it
    to the oven
a cemetery from the 1700s and 1800s
humble pie
making stained glass
three essentials for happiness: something
    to do, someone to love, something to
    hope for
good ol' Vaseline
rainbow-colored fires
the cusp of adolescence

loose strands of hair
writing old friends about new plans
avalanches that are harmless
flying with a tailwind
10 more minutes when you need it
hardware stores with an inexhaustible
    supply of eminently useful items
socks snuggling up to each other in a
    drawer
your first bicycle
when the fourth wheel on a shopping
    cart starts cooperating with the other
    three
potted lemon trees
everyday objects repurposed
feeling like life is worth it
"Dem Bones" (Bible camp song)
a relish tray with a Cheddar spread and
    sweet-and-sour cucumbers
no more tuition or student loan payments
the clap of thunder
wrapping up in blankets, hopping a sled
    drawn by jingle-belled horses, and
    gliding under the stars to a little cabin
the applause of an audience
when you start wanting to eat breakfast
    outdoors in the sunshine
a story that has been handed down
    through your family for generations
windblown hair

rolling suitcases
soft breezes, longer days, lightning bugs,
    and fireworks
hoop earrings
baking in a brick oven
train stops
love
pre-Christmas hustle and bustle
a quaint fishing village of tiny gold-hued
    houses on narrow cobbled streets
magic tricks
Thoroughbred racing
bouncing back
luxuriating in an unhurried morning bath
the dance you perform when a rubber
    band is pointed at you
monkey business
grouping pure white candles in the center
    of a table wreath of pinecones,
    heather, or moss
Shake 'n Bake's combination of flour, oil,
    sugar, mustard, onion, beet, caramel,
    and secret herbs and spices
weeping willows talking of spring
a calendarium
things not always being what they seem
van Gogh's manic skies
biking a railroad trail
putting two and two together
a minor problem

blood banks

fishermen's boats cutting patterns in the sun-gilded water

getting a library card

never forgetting the creation of a special moment

the groceries staying upright when your car turns a corner

burning an orange peel to cover bad cooking smells

mind-mapping

the colors of the rain forest

meditation in a state of activity being a thousand times more profound than that in a state of quietude

operator assistance

fresh water

comfy clothes

sun brightening the brick wall of a house

the young, restless ocean

the clop of horses' hooves

telling spooky stories

great sports comebacks

a bulldozer ride for a child

stone benches

grains of sand viewed through a microscope

margaritas with salt rims

soap carving

pewter, faience, or Dutch delftware

nighttime outdoor parties

flopping in the hammock for a snooze
   before dinner

making confetti with a paper shredder

Charlie Brown's Christmas tree

softening your skin with cocoa butter

summer melons

sheets and pillowcases to dream on

the hairy woodpecker and boreal owl in
   old-growth trees

salad dressing shaken in a cruet

anything or anyone that is on time

bee-drone days and firefly nights

rediscovering croquet

marionette and mime performances

after the beach, taking an outdoor shower
   à deux

a good loser

purchasing a yard of lavender ribbon to
   tie up poems

I.D. pictures

watching a leaf descend

light and tender baked doughnuts,
   brushed with butter and rolled in
   cinnamon sugar

babies eating Cheerios

saying grace softly at the table

swapping fried-chicken recipes over the
   backyard fence

Irish coffee glasses

downward-facing dog in yoga
helicopter sightseeing
pockets crammed with treasures
scientific gadget catalogs
brand-new Ticonderoga pencils
neatly pressed pants
things that come naturally
baby shoes
geraniums in earthenware pots vying
for light
a flower-laden outdoor bar
a stereographic PanoPlanet, multiple
photos to form a 360-degree
panorama of a particular scene
the Four Noble Truths
architects and builders
hottles, glass beverage servers with
black-rimmed neck and cap
learning to swan-dive
baking tiles for the oven
seafood Newburg in patty shells
throwing food pieces into the fire for
scent and color
not staying home alone on Halloween
the apple of your eye
a sink cabinet with a cistern pump
walking to the beach in the morning
going to a palm reader or having your
tea leaves read
a tipple of port

Swiss Army knives, especially the Giant
     with 87 implements
the take-a-penny tray
writing poetry that no one will see
rearranging furniture
painstakingly stuffing the unconscious
     full of facts, impressions, concepts,
     and an endless series of conscious
     ruminations and attempted solutions
tattersall shirts with bow ties
repotting your plants
old-fashioned striped brown bags
Chanel No. 5 cologne
having an avocation
liking others, accepting others, laughing
     with others
research design
a computer's soothing hum
when a snowstorm is abating and the
     setting sun is peeking through low-
     lying clouds
panel quiz shows
owning a watertight car
being caught up with work
banzai, meaning, "May you live 10,000
     years!"
families who summer in the Hamptons,
     the Vineyard, and Nantucket
the suck of a pump
rare moments of true quiet

clothes you pick out as presents from
    parents or relatives
nighty-nights and goodnights
staying in the theater because your date
    wants to watch the credits
a Western Civ. class
Encyclopaedia Britannica on the
    bookshelf
winter vacation kits
wastepaper baskets
cinnamon sugar or maple sugar toast
love light
the flawed process of recollection
making up a guest bed
the ever-changing cards kids collect
searching for pumpkin perfection
paying off a loan or credit card
the Perseids meteor shower
spotting undercover or hidden
    police cars
tissues in every room
spring weekend at college
the icing on carrot cake
academic freedom
birds doing morning "errands"
making sure all the doors are locked
a port-of-call
seeing cows milked, chicks hatch, and
    lambs drink from a bottle
standing up straighter

recognizing how your words affect others

learning things together

a string of Christmas lights that keeps
    changing color

red convertible Alfa Romeo Spiders

keeping fresh flowers by your bed, fresh
    herbs in the kitchen

a fascinating face on the train

comfortable, stretchy clothes

assorted papers in assorted colors

missing someone but knowing you'll
    be together soon

support hose

snappy comebacks to "Shut up"

mulching leaves with a lawn mower

cuticle scissors

the smell of a coffee can opening

fireside pine benches

a vote of confidence

anti-inflammatory medicine

cozy mealtimes

working too hard and getting paid for it

a small orchestra playing for a poolside
    buffet at noon

meanwhile, back at the ranch . . .

spray cologne in your sneakers

beta waves

Everybody mambo!

a slightly stale doughnut, split, sprinkled
    with water, then toasted and buttered

creating a pleasing little surprise for your
partner

the patter of rain

counting down the days to an event

pie-baking contests

self-reliance, strength, pride, and a
romantic vision of life

recreational vehicles plastered with
state and national park decals and
American flags

large colonial fireplaces

finding a purpose

discovering a secret country lane or
peaceful bend in the river

how crazy you were during your college
years

e pluribus unum: out of many, one

the soft splat of snow falling

a cheese board

easily resealed bags

the sharp folds of an elegant fan

making meringue

a ballet leap with the appearance of
being suspended in midair

an old soul

the clinking of ice in a glass

Big Macs

happy hour with former coworkers

renting a small airplane

letting the breezes blow through

delight at the prospect of a new day,
a fresh try, one more start

Big Night (movie)

taking a cooking class together

a silly bubble of anticipation

editing a résumé/CV

remembering the punch line

dancing when you are home alone

faded palaces

Bic pens

a seahorse in an aquarium

Athens marble

jazz percussionists

Christmas celebrated with fireworks

a snow softball

Newport, Rhode Island, in a sleeting
rainstorm

exploring the intricate possibilities of
idleness

Bengay muscle rub

yellow being the most visible of all the
colors in the spectrum

getting up at the cusp of morning

a waterfall wearing a rainbow tiara

a reprieve

sturdy, flat-heeled shoes

having no concern for time, free of the
passions and troubles of the soul,
experiencing something like calm in
the face of things and of oneself

walking around ladders

lonely French fries at the bottom of a fast-food bag

"top ten" and "best of" lists

an Italian coffee press

reading the textbook

a nice comedy

encouraging your children to be creative

the snapping of trodden twigs

making a point without making an enemy

Nebraska: midpoint between the Atlantic and Pacific oceans, cowboys, Herefords, cornfields, Arbor Day

bubble-top buffet servers with hinged lids

lifting your slush-and-snow spirits

oshibana: pressed flowers on rice paper

ridged pasta with a meat sauces, smooth-surfaced pasta with cream or cheese sauces

wallpapering done by a professional

galactic events

being lovey-dovey

magazines in the checkout lane

the sun gently illuminating shades of a verdant wild marsh

a bird catching a fish

onions keeping best when roped and hung in a dry, cold room

stet written in the margin

driving up to a window and being handed
a hamburger and fries
photographing children playing
miniature pinball machines
the speaker of the house
the centrality of the observer's position
being in someone else's wedding party
a sunflower nodding
spotted sandpipers with long bills and legs
Barbie's Dream House and car
cruise control
coin purses
independent bookstores
a room with an old cannonball bed, a
steamer trunk, and a view of Mount
Washington
block-party potlucks
a beer sampler of 4-ounce glasses
a 19th-century pioneer fur-trading post
and gold-mining boomtown
shell-framed mirrors
a distracter, one of the incorrect answers
presented as a choice in a multiple-
choice test
a hot shower after a long trip
closing your eyes and thinking
"black velvet"
waiting by candlelight for a special
person
coed dorms

riding mailboats to remote islands
Sunday afternoon cooking
feng shui
multicolored plastic paper clips
periodicals reserved for bathroom readings
pork belly
tall booths in restaurants
freshly vacuumed carpet or floors
deciding when to bluff
when they replenish the cafeteria food
    right before your turn in line
a box of candy with a guide to what's
    what
meditating in predawn stillness
opening stuck windows
the early, dry dark of an October Saturday
    evening
asking yourself whether you're really
    hungry
swirls of butter in a tub
the tinkling chorus of handbells
"Genius is 1 percent inspiration
    and 99 percent perspiration."
    (Thomas Edison)
living in grace
a wish
an orchestra pit or loft
a studio in a farmhouse on a peninsula
children spinning dreidels
anime hair and eyes

exploring a city at a browser's pace

your underlip

analyticalness

shrink-wrap you can open easily

turning off all the lights during a
thunderstorm

a tutorial when you need it

finding a café, having a cup of coffee and
a snack, then organizing your purse
and cell phone

an armchair in the sun

a gray flannel skirt and navy blazer

lots of books, a good bed lamp, vases of
flowers in the room

isolated country estate atmosphere

foam bath toys

the joy and contentment of listening to
favorite music

brightening someone's day

wearing your new outfit

"When any real progress is made,
we unlearn and learn anew
what we thought we knew before."
(Henry David Thoreau)

a trip to the old neighborhood

the sweet and simple indulgence of an
afternoon nap

sewing name tags on clothes

taking an art appreciation course at a
museum

good solid outdoor exercise or yardwork
the gurgle of running water
Puccini and pasta
your first royalty check
pushing car lighters in
Arkansas strawberries
the point on a potato chip where it breaks
    off and stays behind in the dip
suction cups on bath mats
a thing whose name one forgets,
    does not know, or prefers not
    to mention
Post-its
the ultimate answer to life, the universe,
    and everything in *The Hitchhiker's
    Guide to the Galaxy* (book)
climbing Mount Katadhin
"Rubber Duckie," sung by Ernie
    (Jim Henson)
reflection and reasoning
parasol-sheltered tables
yellow bug lights
spotless chef's whites
GPS in your car and on your phone
white shutters
attempted feedings of children
reading body language
The Graduate (movie)
envisioning your retirement
the desired result on a pregnancy test

poached salmon served with sour cream
  sauce and topped with feathery,
  fresh dill
weather maps
imagined future events
equal rights
painting on a cliffside easel
play being purest relaxation
namelings, people having the same name
when someone vacates a great parking
  spot just as you are pulling in
Too busy? Delegate or organize. No
  money? Borrow or work an extra
  job. Not enough time? Get up earlier
  or stay up later. Don't know enough?
  Take classes.
a landmark East Coast town house
round pancake turners
the piping of a piccolo
bulkie rolls
the life sciences
bobblehead dolls
thirsty plants
what you can learn from the
  Food Network
grown-ups with kids' imaginations
Oklahoma: cattle, football, oil
crisp, leaf-scented air
two odd friends
aging well

the tallest Christmas tree that will fit in
    your living room
knowing the style for a business letter
a friend calling to say, "You did great!"
cash refunds
swinging by the newsstand before work
carpooling
pickles sliced flat for sandwiches
being house-proud
surf culture
proverbs
the fireside being the tulip bed of a
    winter day
bread age by twist tie: Monday = Blue,
    Tuesday = Green, Thursday = Red,
    Friday = White, Saturday = Yellow
a director's cut
"stolen" time
a handy first-aid manual
vein distribution in a maple leaf
creamy garlic salad dressing
finding a taxi in a downpour
all-star games
after-shower cologne
an ice halo with two sun dogs
frost whitening lawns
riding your bike to work
not paying attention to stupid questions
star sapphires
wren houses

a dimly lit room with candles flickering in
red jars

"Keep calm and put your jammies on."

Tao Te Ching

egg salad sandwiches on toast

when you know someone well enough to
go into his/her fridge without asking

the newspaper or magazine at the top of
the stack that everyone passes over,
believing the ones beneath are better

throwing a roof party

requesting information on courses

reading actual handwritten notes in a
cookbook with all the stains and the
wrinkles, marginalia more valuable
and interesting than the recipes

pastry chefs

wide-swinging skirts

getting up when the alarm goes off

parents who inspire their children

speaking up at a meeting

"flats" track shoes

going to an observatory on a star-filled
night

young, spring-grown, just-picked radishes

acclimating oneself to a cold swimming
pool, one body region at a time

a mug's handle, the ear

the white fluff of cattails

sleeping gerbils

workers setting up umbrellas on an
     outdoor restaurant's patio
when a cop finally passes you after
     following you for a long time
trees whispering
aphorism, the residue of complex
     thoughts filtered down to a single
     metaphor
Ordinary, Kentucky
what out-of-towners come to your town
     or region for
seasoning salt: a mixture of salt, pepper,
     garlic, onion, and other spices
calling a friend to meet at the last minute
     and she/he is free and on her/his way
meeting someone who met someone you
     admire
the momentary confusion in a dog whose
     owner has faked throwing a ball
wisps of hair turning up
awesome abandoned places
corrugated cardboard
buying shoes for kids
movie theaters
fireside chats
salt marshes
flexible, bendy straws
a ride on a hay wagon drawn by a pair of
     Belgian draft horses
the beach in winter

someone who reminds us that we are
    not alone
where berries lie in hidden clusters, the
    scent of leaves and ripened fruit
    filling the air
belief in a non-physical entity, the soul
Mississippi: antebellum mansions, magnolia
    trees, shrimp boats, pecan trees
airplane rides
easy-to-read labels
schools for bartending, butlership, fly-
    fishing, clowning, race-car driving
cultivating an open mind
the main arteries of town
butterflies lighting on the rim of a pitcher
the cool, shimmering mist that fishermen
    know on inland lakes
reaching out to another for comfort
learning to enjoy something without
    having to own it
climbing a tall white pine tree
orange crates
a bird teaching a chick to fly
getting somewhere on time
when a baby holds your finger
striped cooks' aprons
living within your income
coat hooks in schoolrooms
waiting for the hidden scene after the
    movie credits roll

porcupine quills

capturing a moment

plenty of ice in the freezer

the intoxicating smell of bacon frying in
the morning

winter scents

the Star of David

cleaning off your desk and buying
new file folders

etched-glass partitions

reading all of Bill Bryson's books

people who don't say "Everything turns
out the way it is supposed to" when
they really don't know that

fireflies winking their undecipherable
messages

a hot baked potato at a restaurant

trestle beds

a quieter happiness

the evolution of a child's vocabulary

a straight black skirt

extra effort always making a difference

determining PSI in basketballs and tires
by feel

hailing a taxi

electric clothes steamers

gambrel-roofed houses

Serengeti lions

merriment, delightful conversation,
toasts, speeches, sharing, kinship

seeing the person in the car next to you
singing along to the radio at the top of
his or her lungs

donating five things you don't need

finding two good reasons to do something

sugar and creamer sets

kitchen parties

an original 1958 blond ponytailed Barbie
Doll

the Winter Palace of Russia

floor mats vacuumed, nothing under the
seats, no dust on the dashboard, no
smudges on the windows

aspen-covered mountains in golden and
amber hues against a backdrop of
dark green fir, spruce, and pine

raised, prominent cheekbones

the exercise of writing things down,
forcing you to pay attention and to
remember

realizing that a well-loved children's
book contains sophisticated
humor, symbolism, or elements of
foreshadowing that you missed when
you were growing up

flickering candlelight

staring out at calm water

dramatic shadows of the descending sun

a backup plan

buying classic clothes

shopping on Christmas Eve

a sacred roof garden

keeping a few little pots of herb butter in
the refrigerator

when you send a text message to
someone and he or she sends one to
you simultaneously

an Italian leather box

peanut brittle

cupholder cuisine

the word *heinie*

New Mexico's state vegetables: the chile
and frijole

a youthful old age

apprenticeship and internship

saving one last treat for the end of
vacation

Kentucky: bluegrass, the Derby,
limestoned valleys, Cumberland Gap

an open tennis court

the ship being absolutely tight before it is
launched

the meaning of existence

cleaning a bike

"All that mankind has done, thought,
gained, or been: it is lying as in magic
preservation in the pages of books."
(Thomas Carlyle)

kids: a very sweet lesson in enjoying life

the lotus position

frost-edged grass blades shimmering in an incredible variety of patterns

molcajete, an authentic Mexican mortar and pestle

blue inlets and crystal creeks

pausing 60 seconds before answering a question

warm cookies and cold milk

muskrat houses

a winter festival of lights

Grandma's meat loaf recipe

feelings of security

the silver screen

Lincoln Memorial, Washington, D.C.

the silent wish you make

being sesquilingual (knowing one and a half languages)

Babar the elephant

complete indifference

digging out a piece of lawn and putting in a garden

the memory of a spring afternoon

people who wear sunglasses at night

the nickname "Gloves"

a beaver dam

apples and bananas in caramel sauce

squirrels darting away with treasure

keeping a sketch pad next to the bed

master keys

library research

scrub oak woods

your demographic group

the Marx Brothers' real names: Julius (Groucho), Arthur (Harpo), Leonard (Chico), Herbert (Zeppo), and Milton (Gummo)

the cocktail party phenomenon where we are able to listen to one person while in a roomful of noise and people

the gypsum sand dunes of White Sands National Monument, moved by the steady southwest winds

the first Harry Potter movie (2001)

strolling a greenhouse for inspiration

mindful fun

turning a Master's into a Ph.D.

reading quietly together

making a leap of faith

cinnamon sticks

silverware bags

never postponing till tomorrow what can be done today

shatterproof bottles

knit-purl combinations

an herb-laced frittata

a bucketful of natural-wood kitchen utensils

peace buttons

inviting your kid to lunch

your new happy place

oiling squeaky things
a tatami used as a bulletin board
hachure in drawing
abracadabra in an inverted pyramid amulet
beamed ceilings
receiving a fabulous gift from the person
    you love
canned soups
Nevada: alkali flats, yucca, sagebrush,
    Las Vegas, silver
upper-crust restaurants
meeting a sports hero
a willow leaf fully grown: a long, slender
    parcel of chlorophyll
being blessed
a first music lesson
one who makes the best of it when he/she
    gets the worst of it
buying new shoes for your sport
birthday banners
the sound of elevator bells, shoppers'
    sighs, and Muzak
the harmless garter snake
copycat recipes
the moon-baying of hounds
the inn dock
stained-glass window and mandala
    coloring books
hibachi cooking
a core asset

suggestions for romantic evenings
words that are marzipan to the tongue
promissory notes
cats basking on the windowsill
"All systems go!"
risotto fritters
onion-skin paper
a fluffy quiver of folded wings
"Seek knowledge to plan, enterprise
    to execute, honesty to govern all."
    (Barkham Burroughs)
all the tiny bumps that make up a basketball
going-out-of-business sales and auctions
listening to someone describe something
    that makes him or her happy
luxuriating with supplies of soaps, body
    lotions, and powders
aged cheese
a super salesperson's spiel
a sense of competence
beef kabobs
heart pacemakers
a blonde moment
older, atmospheric bars
using a paint roller
your favorite word
the minor percentage of the world's
    coupons that are actually used
not being known as grouchy or mean—
    just quiet sometimes

hard cheeses

crossing oneself

a window seat and snacks on the train

dried bouquets of hydrangea, statice,
    baby's breath

not-fit-for-man-nor-beast February nights

Dutch doors

a serious present for a birthday—like
    a desk

the quiet presence of cats

sharing popcorn

sidewalk cheese fries in large paper cups

two boughs crossed in the woods, playing
    backward and forward upon one
    another in the wind

the distance from your elbow to your
    wrist equaling the length of your foot

the irresistible fragrance of toasting bread

running over a piece of lint a dozen times
    while vacuuming, continuing to give
    the vacuum a "chance"

flattering makeup

being as idle as a languid brook

winning a duel

stonewall-lined cow lanes

"Thursday's child has far to go."

coming in out of the rain

real-time information in Wikipedia

conical evergreens

rough beams and fieldstone fireplaces

materials of biological origin occurring
within the Earth's crust that can be
used as a source of energy: coal,
petroleum, natural gas, oil shale,
bitumen, tar sand, and heavy oils
picking the right lane, for once, in a
traffic jam
individual mini crocks
an apartment cook-in
holding hands on the way home from a
concert
kick lines
the neon lights of Hong Kong
ZIP codes
the whistle of the ferries
size 12 women's feet
band rings
confectionery
humorous phone calls
your first paycheck at a new job
opera houses
anticipating vacations
eyeteeth
a strategy for answering SAT questions
"Dr. Livingstone, I presume." (Henry
Morton Stanley)
cool lakes
news conferences
the Dewey Decimal system
snowshoe travel

last summer's shells from the beach
lime marshmallow salad
the feeling of satin
short-sheeting a bed
chimney corners
ravioli cutters
tugs at your scalp when your hair is being
    braided
Jerome Lemelson, the inventor of the
    Walkman, bar code technology,
    the camcorder, and more
creating a romantic picnic from a local
    farmers' market
opening an encyclopedia to a random
    page and reading everything on that
    page
wild blueberries blanketing coastal Maine
young people's concerts
the magic of play in a relationship
the seven holes in a Ritz cracker
a cat peeking at you
the plastic tray used to organize and
    separate silverware
ambling through the best boutiques
finding a way around roadblocks
the overlapping smells of a culinary
    symphony
the steady rhythm of paddling
getaway cars with empty gas tanks
kid gloves

a storm sheathing every cable of the
    Mackinac Bridge in glittering ice,
    making it a silver harp playing the
    music of the wind
tangerine beef and white rice
shallow bowls holding closely clipped
    blossoms
weekend sailors
when the person ahead of you pays your
    toll
startling clarity at 4 a.m.
losing yourself in the ebb and flow of
    serious reflection, neurons humming,
    without letting your attention drift to
    a screen
taking a walk in the rain
a mountain's screes
beginning to feel the faint touch of
    autumn's brush
the days of penny arcades
enough time to do the job right
eating pepperoni out of the package
flight suits
the Acropolis
organizing your goals
planting corn, raising corn, flailing corn
the Great Wall
fruits of the earth
American humor
a mandala's intricate concentric pattern

warming winter meals
open house in a new home
mini tubs of margarine
a sculpture garden
food delivery in a snowstorm
a vacation from buying stuff
fields of June daisies
the importance of turning work into play
the way peanut butter spreads
The Cat in the Hat (Dr. Seuss book)
growing mellow, not hard and brittle
sparkly pom-poms
a booth for quiet cell-phone talking
    between flights
home weather stations
tiny leaves drooping on soft stems, too
    young to hold up their heads
feeding kittens
removing makeup
a bumper sticker on a Dunkin'
    Donuts employee's car that
    says "Lil' Munchkin"
watching the ocean change its moods
living as a free spirit
a blank check
joys and vicissitudes
high-energy slapstick humor
trying again later
coffee fundamentals: proportion, grind,
    water, freshness

an icy diamond-powdering of stars
flaky and nicely browned pastry
theme restaurants for kids
double mattresses on the floor
Art Garfunkel and Paul Simon
streaked hair
springtime in the Rockies
your mom's shredded wheat
littleneck clams on a bed of ice
the word *nincompoop*
fairy tales
a nonclandestine meeting at a hotel
tortoiseshell or wooden combs
outlawing gerrymandering
putting on boots and tramping through
wet fields and woods to remind
yourself of all the things that were
buried or forgotten through the
winter
helping with the farm chores: haying,
milking, grooming the horses
golden lockets
just a moment
an express lane
two-person tents
"May your trails be crooked, winding,
lonesome, dangerous, leading to
the most amazing view. May your
mountains rise into and above the
clouds." (Edward Abbey)

white frame houses in tiny hamlets
Dudley Do-Right and Nell Fenwick (*The Rocky and Bullwinkle Show* cartoon)
keeping a journal of personal definitions and interesting concepts
grocery shopping early in the morning
self-awareness and self-discovery
We Bought a Zoo (movie)
avoiding drama
Hollywood love lives
ice-skating at midnight
Arm & Hammer baking soda
elephants sliding down a slope for their morning bath
the chowder kettle
addressing a golf ball
categorization projects
a screened porch on your house
what you enjoy about yourself
dressing to the max and flirting
dancing at a Cajun festival
an individual sconce to illuminate an eating booth
when people drive you home and wait until you unlock the door before driving away
free stuff from a hotel
spring salads
the smell of chalk and pencil shavings
unlocked gridlock

making decisions
devil's food
the cinema
an all-night vigil of pleasure
Julia Child's home kitchen
stepping out of your life in order to put
    things in perspective, solving knotty
    problems by directing your gaze at
    something or someone else
jumping off the bandwagon
"You name it!"
master lists
caring for new woodwork
little, round ball candles
professional landscaping
hot appetizers
the ketchup that collects at the lip of the
    bottle
waking up to a snowstorm or brilliant
    sunshine in winter
stomping in mud puddles
white 100 percent cotton sheets
Curious George
mellowed red brick walls
French rolling pins
melon or grapefruit served with honey
    instead of sugar
"Never mind!"
painting yourself accidentally
the glow of the holidays

the gravity-defying Round-Up fair ride
a cache of Moleskine notebooks
a blank slate
hot prepared chili on a hot dog
expecting nothing
The Importance of Being Earnest (play)
Cheesequake or Dicktown, New Jersey
recipe-card libraries
the ability to admit a weakness
surprising someone with his or her
    favorite sandwich
the stillness of granite
Lake Michigan's shoreline
sucking in air so crisp and clean that you
    think you have never really had the
    experience of breathing before
a room to retreat to for listening to music,
    puttering, looking through books, and
    clipping magazines
teaching someone how to use a thesaurus
hiring a charter boat
when the pancakes you make look like
    the ones pictured on the box
cultivating mindfulness and loving-
    kindness throughout each day
when your adult child tells you he respects
    you as a person and considers you to
    be one of his best friends
copper-bottomed pans
generous dollops of humor

lowering your voice when you feel it is
    about to rise
ensuring there will be at least one slice of
    banana for every spoonful of cereal
pasta with prosciutto and peas
friendship cards
beef on a stick and chicken fingers
someone saying, "Well done!"
running mates
commonsense folk sayings
having one child who plays drums and
    one who plays guitar
riding a bicycle long distances
on a rainy evening, continuing writing
    your magnum opus
the taste of vacuum coffee on a sunlit
    bank or sandbar
Chuckles candy
hearth glow
believing that what you think about
    is different from what others
    think about—a struggle going on
    inside to find some sort of creative
    or spiritual or aesthetic way of
    seeing the world and organizing
    it in your head
reincarnation or rebirth
toy soldiers
old friends to help us grow old
the exact time you were born

squash players
cushioned tile
the nickname "Peaches"
the exhausted clothes in the hamper
getting your act together
one perfect rose
nutmeg graters
direct/nonstop cross-country flights
doing things right the first time
books of facts
plus-fours golf pants
handmade ski sweaters
realizing your child is a good reader
a factlet, piece of trivia
seasonable weather
letting your hair grow
in-ground pools
Egypt's Valley of the Kings
Angora rabbits
singing in cars
cell-phone insurance
the full moon rising when the sun sets
waking up with a cat
"It is the greatest of all mistakes to do
        nothing because you can only do
        little. Do what you can." (Sydney
        Smith)
tractor pulls
lanes that lead to the sea and the
        rockbound coast

lake steamers
Dutch tulip bulbs
parents' weekend at college
warm fluffy clothes straight from
    the dryer
the U.S. Marine Corps' Silent Drill Team
"Tennis, anyone?"
the band coming out for one last song
clumps of blackberry brambles heavy
    with ripening fruit
dribbling a basketball like Meadowlark
    Lemon
an accomplishment that is all yours
the dark line of a storm on the horizon
    growing wider and closer
ordering dessert
building permanent bookcases
visiting a Nativity scene
comparing books to their movies
learning the harmonica
the tiny fragments of toast left behind
    in the butter
drivers yielding to other drivers
tree-sitting
prairie dogs kissing
asking simple questions
government employees
Midnight in Paris (Woody Allen movie)
a team coming through a paper hoop at
    the game

antique violins
being able to draw a fleur-de-lis
catnip mousies
the sun shining through a blue haze
petting a horse
tiny bird footprints
cranberry-orange muffins
a stream laughing as it tickles its own
	snowy banks
sledding on the lawn
easily slipping the fitted sheet over
	each corner of the bed
being kinder than necessary
pince-nez glasses
the possibility of life on Mars
your child securing a good summer job
the color of bread crust
safety razors
weathered towers on high hills
defying gravity
tiny spring peeper frogs
a baby grand piano in the front parlor
thick slices of eggplant
utility stools
taking fewer things seriously
unwrapping sandwiches
dreaming on the riverbank
a living room's litter of unwrappings on
	Christmas or birthdays
a really cool crib design

a bowl of tiny mandarin oranges
freedom of the press
hot, gooey chocolate chip cookies
a knife block keeping everything safe
    and organized
men's ties
a broad porch, ideal for rocking
butter-basted fried eggs
a lively discussion group
college-age road trips
checking the faces of departing
    moviegoers in an attempt to
    determine the quality of the film
a half bath in the basement
using your unique skills to help others
a hot fudge sundae: the perfect combo of
    hot and cold
finishing a novel that has on the last page
    THE END
that there is more to cooking and baking
    than simply opening a box or
    reheating a meal
buying a T-shirt in five colors
green grass reaching for sunlight through
    cracked pavement and vacant-lot
    rubbish
satchel bags
rosti: partially cooked potatoes formed
    into broad pancakes and fried until
    golden

stretch pants

collar buttons

Jean-François Champollion, decipherer of the Rosetta Stone

anniversary telegrams

viewing everyday surroundings with a tourist's eye

Charleston, flamenco, go-go, and jive dancing

when blush was called rouge

baby terrariums

a roll of quarters for the casino

weeding and grooming the garden

being a Buddha

peppermint extract

Cape Cod cranberries

sitting on the porch in cold autumn weather

being a novice hiker

sautéed Canadian bacon

wedding cake

Irish setters

a gray fuzzy sweater and gray satin skirt

watching a big moon skim in and out of the clouds, smelling the thick, fragrant country air

batting cages

the position of point guard

keeping in step

chrome-and-glass tables

bouquets of roses wrapped in white paper
        and tied with luscious red ribbons
potato bread
chestnut trees, heavy with blooms
antiquated customs
a treat for the house
proudly wearing a wedding band
an ivory slipper chair
horticultural techniques
brevity and conciseness
brand-new homes
dynamic workplaces
ocean wading
getting skates sharpened
a fix-it shop that goes to heroic measures
        to fix things
remembering when phone exchanges all
        had names
the etcetera of a list
figuring out the F buttons on your
        computer
someone calling and inviting you to lunch
choosing a Christmas tree
organization of errands
tobogganing
thick, golden curried potato soup
long-stemmed lilies
letting the crowd follow
thick fur on the bottom of rabbits' feet
endless excuses not to work

getting a cast or braces taken off
Hush Puppies shoes
something that just feels right
taking a bowl of berries or thick, fruity
    yogurt out to the patio or front stoop
glimpsing a horizon through a cluster
    of trees
cheap eats
waterfalls: ledge, plunge, horsetail,
    cascade, staircase, cataract,
    segmented, tide fall
big joys and small pleasures
farm-style picnics featuring chicken,
    turkey, beef, fresh garden salads and
    vegetables, homemade cakes and
    pies, relishes, and potato salads
food imaginatively prepared and eaten in
    good company
an entourage
dietary fiber
befriending a linebacker
tasting a dish while it's cooking
the Man in the Moon
toasty warmth
the Heart Sutra
beach plum jam
arable land
watching bartenders who work really fast
curious and expectant travelers
TTFW: too tacky for words

a plate filled with food set in front of a
     hungry teenager

a riverboat restaurant decorated with lots
     of sparkling white lights

funnel cakes, deep-fried to a golden
     brown and served hot with a coating
     of powdered sugar

heads and tails

a crisp, perfectly salted French fry

woven straw mats

chautauquas

the miniature bells of white lily-of-the-
     valley

foals and horses

the special blimp camera for nationally
     televised sporting events

meat-and-three restaurants

George Harrison and Ringo Starr of
     the Beatles

a cocoon hanging by a silk thread

a vandyked grapefruit

shocks of corn

barn swallows swooping

an October sun peeking into the car
     windows

broiled mahi mahi with mango

going where there's still room

falling asleep to the sound of surf
     crashing as you nestle in your
     campsite

when the worst does not happen
the way a bird's wing has the same basic
    bone structure as the human arm
    and hand
lawn-cutting, garden-tending, house-
    tidying chores
avocado in salad
laundering your money, literally
manicotti, the pillows of pasta stuffed
    with cheese and covered with
    bubbling red sauce
hybrid cars
the beauty of the 10,000 things around you
maiden names
Rodgers and Hart songs
anything that increases our empathy for
    other human beings
valuable journeys, which are not easy
the day when you met your best friend
a shakin' paint-mixing machine
the ballot box
rumpusing around on rainy days
a wagon wheel
wearing safety glasses outside lab class
renting a car at the airport and using GPS
    to find your way to a new town
fresh blueberry sauce to serve over a
    favorite ice cream
summer homes in Vermont
flirtatiousness

the kind of chocolate cake that
   automatically suggests a glass of milk
naming your rock band
learning the art of compromise
"Open" signs
a mapped but hidden city street
reverie and conversation
old housekeeping books
when you switched from a desktop to a
   laptop
R.O. Blechman's drawings
strong French-roasted coffee and hot milk
   poured at the same time into large
   breakfast cups
inviting someone special to tell you a
   secret wish
sleepy eyes
sawdust floors
blizzard lights on the car
dogs at field hockey practice
learning a new dance
the Parthenon
country music
paper dolls
rainwater on green leaves
obtaining that which is elusive
being charming
a black lava–strewn coast
trainee hats
the shortest distance between two points

shining indoor plants' leaves with
    mayonnaise
mistakes: portals of discovery
cutting bangs
working with a tablet in a wireless
    environment
refinishing furniture
a school dance
the awesome achievement of the building
    of Inca structures at extremely high
    altitudes
hot avgolemono soup for your cold
space-saving ideas
Wisconsin and Iowa prairie
sports trophies
coffee "with socks on" (with cream)
oatmeal days
the average of 1,800 thunderstorms
    going on in the world at all times
white bread or multigrain?
slipcovers and futon covers
a life-size drawing or representation
divvied-up pie
micro-massage products
platinum credit cards
flower arrangements scenting a room
"the hots"
remembering being picked up and rocked
    to sleep in someone's arms, then
    carried up to bed

cheese shops
backroading
mouthwatering descriptions
unfinished kindergarten blocks
five people reading one newspaper
snowboarding in Vermont
meeting deadlines
Limoges boxes
watching the National Spelling Bee on TV
a game going into overtime
brand-new, unscorched pot holders
smoked chicken
bone-deep contentment
brightening up one's spirits
homemade caramel corn
country house hotels
"smile" buttons
stones swelling and shrinking with the
    changing temperature and humidity,
    the color also varying
cotton towels
ingredients for cooking
real estate
e-cards
The New Yorker magazine
aiming for more quality
smooth, muscular arms
acres of books
"Cat: One hell of a nice animal, frequently
    mistaken for a meat loaf." (B. Kliban)

great luxury

the decision of whether or not to have kids

measuring things

a special coffee shop

true, lasting values

a room filled with candlelight at Christmas

brick streets

slowing down your breathing, visually taking in your surroundings

not expecting too much

a quiet rooster

reading books written by travelers

casual Friday dinners

pumpkin gnocchi

running backs

making sure you have what you need before helping others (e.g., putting on your oxygen mask first)

effortlessness

whistlin' Dixie

breakfasting outdoors in a thatched-roofed restaurant

a great song title

dessert parties

an outside chance

watching your clothes dryer's spin cycle for excitement

a cat running 30 mph

letting someone in line get in front of you
sitting on the grass with a child and
     playing
the Abominable Snowman
wedding gown fittings
a solo vacation
knitting slippers
the spirit of coping well
nicknames
interviews with coaches
the neighborhood spaghetti joint
biding your time
the Cotton and Rose Bowl parades
Halloween smelling of wet, burning
     insides of pumpkins
the 15,000 different kinds of rice that exist
boots for pigs
the age of consent
swing choirs
an unexpected kindness
ceremonial attire
partly cloudy (what we think of as partly
     sunny) 3/8 to 5/8 cloud cover, mostly
     cloudy 6/8 to 7/8 cloud cover, and
     cloudy 8/8
biting a fingernail and it comes off cleanly
aisle seats whenever you travel
seaside amusement parks
sudden darkness
bathroom cups

"I love you more than yesterday, less than
     tomorrow."
the first time you heard the Beatles
pretending to be an Olympic swimmer
the order of probability for throwing dice:
     7, 6, 8, 5, 9, 10, 4, 3, 11, 2, 12
the prospect of learning
Noodle, Texas
baked spaghetti
pancake shops
air fresheners
asking what the future is
birds' mating calls
grass stains that come out of clothes
Holy Communion
the opportunity for a college education
a meatball restaurant
knowing where all your books are
a wheel of Stilton cheese
resort living
a snowman on the football field
"Health, love, wealth, and time to enjoy
     them." (slogan)
airmail stamps and stationery
what you are thinking right now
veils of rain
black-and-white photography
anesthesia
weather satellites
political discussions on breaks and at lunch

starting a kid's savings account
reading a magazine with someone
pullout writing boards on desks
company picnics
unweaving tinsel from tree branches
chilled pears
a California king-size bed
frankfurters
crackle glaze ceramic
Hygiene, Colorado
seventh-grade basketball
any sunny day
a picnic in front of the fireplace
browsing in a toy store
high school sweethearts
squeezed cherries with a scoop of vanilla
    ice cream
getting a foot in the film business
hot days and cool nights
not being typecast
dreams of singing in a club or restaurant
scorching edges of paper for effect
track-and-field days
having your luck suddenly change for the
    better
work shoes
the impact of irrigation
writing your memoirs
a toast rack
the "everybody plays" philosophy

cottontail rabbits
life's great pleasures
bicycling at a state park
charity and thrift shops
Zen, a translation of Chinese meaning
    "quietude," from a root meaning,
    "to see, observe"
devilish grins
steering-wheel covers
eating outside with the smell of the ocean
every day being the happiest of your life
italic writing
your favorite brand of exercise clothes
    and shoes
thistledown tufts riding every gust of wind
pretty or amusing sleep masks for when
    the sun's pouring in
marketing a fad
Wednesday-night TV
lizards scooting
being soothed when awakened from a bad
    dream at 3 a.m.
overnight camping on the gym floor
emerging into sunshine from a tunnel
going for a "walking meal," stopping for
    different courses along the way
book learning
a waterfall cascading amid bright floral
    colors and the sloping greenery of
    wide lawns

chicken wire

hunting for natural-wood sculpture in early morning after a storm or a first frost

a house in the National Register

the "snuggle right in" feeling

carrying only the necessary baggage

the turning earth, the blazing sun, the restless wind

having your hair highlighted

warm pies and spiced whipped cream

getting to McDonald's right when they are switching from breakfast to lunch

becoming transfixed by the movement, sounds, and rhythm of the surf: waves crashing, then gently rolling in and edging back

open-to-the-sky freedom

aardvark, an animal mostly found in the pages of a dictionary

a multicolored handbag

using large scallop shells to serve coquilles St. Jacques, salmon mousse, marinated scallops, or shrimp cocktail

sitting on the roof

coaches all dressed alike

turning the page

slicing through satiny mushrooms

birds on a branch

a bluish haze in the Great Smoky
Mountains National Park, created by
moisture and oils released by the trees
street hockey
an inchworm on an autumn leaf
a four-hankie flick on the Late-Late
cash reserves
baby floodlights
looking for good things in everyone
happy aromas
the warm glow of Sabbath candles
the childhood fun of singsong nursery
rhymes
flat, sharply focused computer monitors
broad purple pools of shadow lying in
every hollow
the global commons
British spellings: centre, colour, flavour,
honour, theatre
the reward of repetition
zigzag weaves
zirconias passing for diamonds
"Happiness is not having what you want,
but wanting what you have." (Rabbi
Hyman Schachtel)
empty crab shells on the beach
being selective
embracing feelings of hopelessness as a
source of mental and spiritual relief
from the stress of constant striving

opening day of the season for the
     ice-cream shop
magnetic letters on the refrigerator
a list being at least four things, a doublet
     for two things, and a tricolon for
     three things
the bulge of athletes' muscles
a wish for adventure
4-H ribbons
wall stenciling
Girl Scout handbooks
belly dancers
the perfume of pines and azalea blossoms
     and fresh-turned earth
hard, young tomatoes
light switches
natural wild mustard
a 6-foot grinder for the Super Bowl party
stargazing
wooden steps
fireworks finales
using Q-tips responsibly
the home-baking enthusiast
construction workers
taking up chess together
coming out of a supermarket in a
     good mood
gloriously satisfying extravagances
hand muffs
a pebble-dash facade

an "invisible fence"
those precious moments when your brain
     feels blank, the gift of being present
     without thoughts running through
     your head
toponyms and their origins
a walk in the country with a friend
appreciating the effort of 12 bees making
     1 teaspoon of honey
Dick Tracy
steak fries
birds huddling on the ground
carol singing, children squealing,
     New Year's toasting
centuries-old dirt lanes leading to hidden
     ancestral homes
forgetting to turn the oven on
books in the bathroom
chewing your food slowly so you can
     savor all the flavors
umami, the fifth taste, found in soy
     products and Asian foods
the first day of September
quiet drives with no radio/CD or cell
     phone allowed
"The early bird catches the worm."
hanging popcorn balls on the tree
the blizzard that hulks beyond the horizon
pineapple juice
crewneck sweaters

"A penny for your thoughts."

when your mom wraps a warm towel
around you when you get out of a
cold lake on a hot day

white elephants

happy children

ink etchings

four-wheel drive in a snowstorm

a Saturday morning with cartoons,
relaxing in pajamas with a bowl
of cereal

baskets filled with fake fruit or bread

eating so much spaghetti that you
cannot move

the Yale libraries, especially Sterling

sometimes just having to say, "What
the hell!"

patio lights

picture-book villages

taking a water taxi

city council meetings

crisp cotton dresses

a string of Greek worry beads

the swish of a silken dress

Neosporin on a cut

floating mollusks, strange fern forests,
huge dinosaurs, flying lizards, and
giant mammals whose bones lay
under the dropped boulders of
vanished continental ice sheets

spending a whole night reading,
    sometimes even alternating books
"We Used to Be Friends" (theme song of
    Veronica Mars, performed by the
    Dandy Warhols)
Aruba coffee, chicory coffee
finding a fort
the spiced aroma from the pickling kettle
    in the rural kitchen
the secrets of closets
enjoying the morning sun on the patio
bonus free throws
being respected for what you do
memories of garden parties and weekends
    by the sea
velvet-starred nights
the thumping of a bass drum
Be Kind to Animals
chaos, a great teacher
averting your eyes
knowing we all want to be happy and
    we're all going to die
rolling hill country
wide beaches
the thunderous drum of the ocean beating
    down on rocks
maple keys
cats' love of fleece
Federalist and Greek Revival houses
a caring doctor

the corrugator on the forehead that
     contracts it into wrinkles and pulls
     the eyebrows together
camping cots
sharing "I have always wanted to" stories
a space heater in your office
when good things happen to people you
     care for
ignorance being bliss sometimes
the first Hot Wheels car, a Chevrolet
     Camaro
playfulness
making up for lost time
layering on favorite old sweaters
taking Sunday papers to the park
top bananas
towel-dried hair
barely sidestepping some dog poo on the
     sidewalk
children who admit their parents are right
     sometimes
the innate and biological capacity of
     humans to understand grammar
air-brushed photographs of you
building a great sand castle
a total sky-opening
     bucketing down of rain
a sleep-and-study loft
living wills
the natural look of yellow face powder

the gift of undivided attention
the first set of new Crayola colors:
  cerulean, dandelion, wild strawberry,
  vivid tangerine, fuchsia, teal blue,
  royal purple, jungle green
party invites
French lace
love and kisses
silver-plated baby mugs
floor pillows
a total eclipse
your website gaining users
digital clocks
thinking to yourself, "I'm so glad I got this
  seat" on the subway or train—and
  feeling relaxed and at ease
cadmium yellow
shuffling cards
the critical period in matrimony being
  breakfast time
buying a painting from a starving artist
educated grace
the first 10 seconds after you turn out the
  lights and wiggle yourself into a good
  sleeping position
phoning home
the ability to cut a piece of cake with
  a little plastic fork on a flimsy
  paper plate while holding a drink
  and napkin

sentences: elastic patterns of linked words
color therapy
old-fashioned iceboxes
being free to change and express yourself
getting a back scratch
Hawaiian shirts
bringing home a surprise from
    a bake shop
Thomas Edison inventions: waxed paper,
    mimeograph, electric light, motion-
    picture camera, dictating machine,
    electric vote recorder machine,
    storage battery, phonograph record,
    electric pen, electric railway car,
    stock ticker, electric railroad signal,
    light socket, light switch
manhandling the "Open here" spout of a
    milk carton so badly that you have to
    resort to using the "illegal" side
disinterest in the race for status
the process of choosing a car
being cool
dark, swarthy types
synthetic airplane pillows and sober navy
    blue scratchy blankets
a Matchbox version of your dream car
refried beans, sour cream, shredded
    cheese, guacamole, diced tomatoes,
    scallions, and black olives
finding the start of a roll of toilet paper

assertiveness

quality time with yourself or others

making an adventurous new ethnic meal

touching toes in bed

seeing city lights from above

the six Gummi Bears' names: Gruffi, Cubbi,
Tummi, Zummi, Sunni, Grammi

great airline snacks

silly season

Thanksgiving Day parades

staying away from anyone named
"Honest John"

bicycle hikes

finding a newspaper someone left on
the train when you were too cheap
to buy one

the lightly sweetened crispiness of
General Tso's chicken nestled in a
bed of flash-cooked broccoli

first-aid kits

cute sneezes

walking a dog by the ocean

waiters smiling when they see you

fresh lemon juice

"saucering" in the snow

nirvana in the Berkshires

servings of local cheese and honey

grilled lamb medallions with apricot sauce

velleity: a mild desire, wish, or urge that is
too slight to lead to action

the theory that the first 12 days after
     Christmas indicate what each month
     in the next year will be like
smoky eyes
being ergonomically correct at the office
wondering why things look the way they
     look, feel the way they feel, how
     they're used and why
the take-your-picnic-indoors plan
the icicle hanging at the eave
"No problem!"
talking to the tiny perforations on a cell
     phone
Murphy's Law
full recoveries when they weren't expected
when all the reference letters for college
     are written
"A wise man will make more opportunities
     than he finds." (Francis Bacon)
a ritual in reminiscence
reading poetry before bed
Kentucky horse-breeding
cubed steak
an entrance to an undersea cave
people zooming on hang gliders
giving yourself the day off
believing as many as six impossible things
     before breakfast (paraphrased, Lewis
     Carroll)
nursery monitors and cameras

the magic workings of a flower, of a
    migrating bird, and man's intellect
the internal treasures that we accumulate
    each year of our lives
mechanical engineering
complimenting a total stranger
maple syrup muffins with maple icing
"Time is money."
seeing amazing choreography
"Monday's child is fair of face."
browsing in cooking supply stores
a parenthesis in time
people who don't "put on airs"
fishing lures
friends spending the night
the national No-Call List to stop solicitor
    phone calls
grungy clothes
the grand total
having a butterfly ride along on your arm
    while you are hiking
absolute revelations
someone fixing something without being
    asked
lounging on the deck
winning an essay contest
Saturday night
spun glass
magic lanterns
Sadie Hawkins dances

finding a path of footprints in the sand at
the beach and following the entire
distance of that person's walk
the interior monologue you experience
when you sit down to write
a small music box that plays *The Blue
Danube* and a tune from *La Traviata*
the numbers 60, 24, and 7 thought to be
magical in the past—influencing the
number of minutes in an hour, hours
in a day, days in a week
asking first
the Rangeley knot on moccasins
big parties with beautiful people
trees' preparations for winter
being alone in a public restroom
soil horizons
knowing what to do in emergencies
neither scurrying nor haste at an early
hour
whoever first thought to eat turtle soup
a ladies' lunch
the world's digital library
the car heater
abandoning all your senses to a field of
wildflowers
entertaining the idea of a career change
sport fishing
the syncopation of a conductor's wand
never stepping into the same river twice

sub shops and fried-clam stands
dog tricks
not begrudging others what you cannot
    enjoy
buying oceanside property
spring-cleaning your computer
when the caffeine kicks in
giving presents to yourself
finding a four-poster at a country auction
a fresh tomato from the garden
planning a cheese plate
roadside rest stops
the slight bending of light as it passes
    the edge of an object, depending
    on the wavelength of light
the notion of time
secret caves
bread factories
swimming a ¼ mile being equal to
    running 1 mile
New York City ballet companies
"Turn Off TV, Turn On Life"
getting a quick answer
starting the coffee machine in the morning
flamboyant typography
glaciers that pour out of the mountains
    like iridescent monsters slithering
    down to the sea
table-hopping at a wedding reception
an air of expectancy

your first love
adventures that don't require equipment
planning your future with the help of a
    Ouija board
the small piece of lid that the electric can
    opener always passes over
December symbols: turquoise or zircon
    birthstones; holly, narcissus, or
    poinsettia
Timbuktu in Mali
optimism you bring to a task
western sundowns
Campbell's tomato soup
writing it down!
the coolth of evening
midday repast
going to the movies in the afternoon when
    you're supposed to be at work
fascination with the Weather Channel
winter forcing you to stay home and get
    acquainted with yourself
drawing a realistic picture
a bandstand on the town green
foods that no one can eat gracefully:
    powdered doughnuts, corn on the
    cob, melting ice cream, barbecue ribs,
    Buffalo wings, a huge slice of pizza
the purr of a kitten
crawling out of a tent on a frosty morning
new sandals

the hearty taste, rich aroma of fresh yeast,
and golden brown crust of bread

finding a hammock and setting out to
be lazy

the grating of a rusty hinge

eminent success

a 5,000-volume library

wearing your favorite outfit on tough days

watching birds

the streetlights of town, like an enchanted
pearl necklace disappearing around a
small hill

seeing someone famous at a baseball
game

sunny weddings

pine-clad peninsulas

when the food you enjoy eating is healthy

a rendezvous

Highway 1 along the Big Sur coast of
California

pocket concerts of jingling keys and
change

downhill racers

being liked by the family of your
significant other

drinking a glass of cold water right after
eating ice cream

Walden by Henry David Thoreau

well-lit rooms

the gift of a sunflower

drawing the curtains on a leaden
     afternoon sky, turning with relief
     to an open fire
for November chills: thick chili, loaves of
     crusty bread, and crunchy crudités
embellishing wild-night-out stories
listening to happy music
when the smell of a good dinner is still
     around for a few hours
projects or activities you are looking
     forward to
setting a trend
working with a new client
Caesar salads
dew-hung spiderwebs
the twirling-fork-in-bowl-of-spoon school
     of spaghetti eating
a TV show worth watching
inserting change in a vending machine
     according to size or value
protozoa and your first microscope
easy-to-peel tangerines
stretch lace
paid internships
tabby cats
cheek-to-cheek dancing
marrying money
the Welcome signs of the states
leaf-fall bringing a crisp scuffling as the
     wind courses the land

bars of late afternoon sunshine
the willingness to do irrational things in
    the pursuit of phenomenally unlikely
    payoffs
cream-soda lollipops
treating yourself to a new purse
marble-topped dressers
finding an Easter egg in your raincoat
    pocket
Frank Lloyd Wright's design of the
    Guggenheim Museum
dressing almost totally in L.L. Bean
busy city life
an accredited school
Heath Bar Crunch ice cream
lake sailing
eating less, chewing more
relief that hard or stressful times are over
an hour to go
job-hunting strategies
melted butter
muddling a lemon to release the essential
    oils
sharp kids
lumps that block the pouring spouts of
    sugar dispensers
library sofas
municipal golf courses
night games
fogbows

squeezing into a booth and squinting at
the small-font menu under the dim
lighting
Arctic hares growing a thicker coat
a song brightening your mood
split Portuguese rolls with butter
the splash of a fish
spending money on things that cultivate
experiences
acting class
mammoth dictionaries
campfire wood
free wireless Internet access
robot servants
the size of fall fashion magazines
the deposit that beats your rubber check
to the bank
taking a weekend trip by yourself
blue collarism
the white tips of a French manicure
the art of verbal embroidery
The IT Crowd (British TV comedy)
cheeks a chipmunk would be proud of
celery and cream cheese
silence after a busy day
the crystal lining of a geode
the adventures of our lives
an unusual setting for a candlelight
dinner
cake stands

"You can't take it with you."
when you get up at 4 a.m. and see how
    many of your neighbors are also
    up at that time
knowing the correct pronunciation
book clubs
hosting a party
a survival kit for someone who is sick:
    favorite magazines, books, remote
    control for the TV, soup, juices, and
    a handmade "feel better" card
cardinals, quail, and robins flitting about
    the rhododendron and mountain
    laurel
supper salads
hanging a mirror to reflect the greenery
    and sunshine of an outdoor view
a motel room with a clean kitchenette
smelling roses in a vase
international cookbooks
having free-and-clear title
tools and workbenches
setting up the bath as a cul-de-sac: a tub
    tray, bookrest, inflatable bath pillow
using TiVo or DVR to catch up with a
    favorite show
watching a late-season game with playoff
    implications
azure skies
limbo contests

hand-hammered cowbells

guides to the best and worst of everything

a cure for a disease

a love you can count on

smokestacks autographing the sky

when the right word comes to mind

agricultural surpluses

cooking a quick dinner for company

piling on the blankets for a good, cozy
night of sleeping

dogs wanting belly rubs

restful sojourns

Halloween masks

when you are watching one of your
favorite movies and you realize you
do not remember how it ends

sweet honesty

Chinese cabbage

running down a beach

country French blue-and-red checks

squirrels in reckless treetop chases

basement swings

eating the chocolate Easter bunny's head
first

a knowledge "adventure"

not standing idly by

meeting a studio mogul on the red-eye
from LA

Egyptologists who are also mystery
writers

Nesselrode pie
warm afghans
learning the silk-screening process
sting, the musical phrase played after a
    joke or skit
exploring neighborhoods in places you
    might want to live
James Taylor (singer)
being the bearer of good news
a box of Lincoln Logs
rocks dashed with sea
pop culture
running a dairy
lightning rods
the Upper Peninsula of Michigan
bringing a cookout down to the beach
"butter" suns
A Hard Day's Night (movie)
a staring contest
wide streets
untangling something
when you go to the movies and there are
    all-new previews
oil-free makeup
salad days
reserved seats
taking your own sweet time
having something bright yellow in your
    room at work
your one great old-reliable cookbook

perfect balance on the subway without
    holding on
bopping in your chair when you hear a
    good song
the stars having a frosty twinkle
taking note of all the interesting things
    you see, hear, smell, etc.
switching places in bed with your spouse
enjoying fall yardwork
rowboats pulled up on a
    sandy beach
the sweet sound of an old violin
when it rains after you exercise
    outside
planning your megahit
honey graham crackers
your first Christmas tree together
finally getting the pebble out of your shoe
the dots between syllables in a dictionary
the annual flip-flop sale at Old Navy
picnic grounds
palindrome: a sentence or group of words
    that reads the same backward as
    forward
Tonka trucks
orange pekoe tea
birch bark
an amazing slot canyon, often less than
    3 feet wide and more than 100 feet
    deep, on the Colorado Plateau

"Love is patient, love is kind."
(Ecclesiastes)
a face without makeup
large Christmas lights on trees outside
a restaurant
electric blankets
the last winter break of your college years
tongue-and-groove walls and ceilings
pork sausage
a successful dry run
inner resources
reading the paper outside on the porch,
curled up in a big old rocking chair
making others curious
eating the first freshly baked cookie from
the oven even though it is way too hot
flagpole-sitting
solar energy
cut and paste
poems carved in monuments
auspices
pizzazz
the voice of your ancestors
real cream—thick, tenderly yellow,
perfectly sweet
getting to work on time
the stirring beat of a fife-and-drum corps
shorelines
cats who love being chased
the chambered nautilus shell

children's mittens saved over the years
and hung on the wall as a collection
of winter memories
dinner for four
patience and fortitude
fashion hindsight
unspoiled beaches, isolated moors, quiet
country lanes
homemade cranberry sauce
washing the car
taking forever to get dressed
rice pudding after Indian food
cotton clouds
self-tanning sprays and lotions
paper baskets of gumdrops, tiny
jellybeans, and heart-shaped
candy wafers printed with words
of affection
searching in cookbooks for something
new for dinner
red suspenders
oak spiral staircases
self-esteem
easy-to-clean slipcovered cushions
taking a child to the zoo or park
Granny Smith, Golden Delicious,
Cortland, McIntosh, and Jonathan
apples
making better choices
Sunday afternoon bowling

a cozy, family-run restaurant

catching a falling leaf to make a wish
    come true or for a day of good luck

tightening the screws in an assembly or
    repair job

using mesquite wood in the barbecue for
    a smoked flavor

getting out of the car and stretching at the
    highway rest stop

defrosting a refrigerator

applying makeup

the red light in the church chapel

wind songs

flowers in an empty mustard or cheese
    crock

following a butterfly

a toasty paved road in August

remembering something you memorized
    long ago

pleasing colors, shapes, textures

being kissy

no longer comparing yourself to others

The Joy of Cooking and *Pillsbury
    Kitchens' Family Cookbook*

running around in circles

teaching a class

corn shucks

the slow lap of water at moored boats

just one day of looking terrific

boxed cake

grosgrain ribbon for bookmarks
faithfulness
carnations with baby's breath
indulging in the rich self-pity of
    believing that nobody can
    possibly understand you
a sunrise with no stage fright
lovestruck porcupines
pastry crimpers
your favorite newspaper columnist
uninhibited statements
being passionately curious
taking yourself to lunch
Christmas tree farmers
those moments of life that are utterly
    simple
trusting the process
being on the first-string team
clipping cartoons to save
forging ahead
lying in a field of soft grass with the wind
    blowing over your body
snacks in the pantry
the countryside bathed in autumn sunlight
a beautiful state of mind
KFC coleslaw
making a documentary
spring rolls
bench saws
a reassuring ritual

The Fabulous Baker Boys (movie)

a chance to sleep in

thirsty children kissing water from a
fountain

grandparents who don't undo years of
parental discipline in one weekend

a pochade box

turkey stuffing

an elegant archway

the concept of the music "mix"

when a cat has seen a dog

schizocarps: the wing-like single seeds
that fall from maple trees

carrying all the groceries
in from the car

stockings hung from the
chimney with care

half-baked people

repurposing churches and
warehouses as housing

making a rubber-band ball

St. Croix, Virgin Islands

gifts wrapped in tissue paper, tied with
red ribbon

the start of a new sports season

not being able to fight sleep on the bus

picking the right direction at a fork in
the road

sirloin, filet, or rib-eye steak with choice
of cut, size, and degree of doneness

beignets: flaky, powdered-sugar pastry
squares
getting the last item on the shelf
a good consolation prize
Toby Tyler (1960 movie)
still finding that screaming into a pillow
is the best stress relief
tranquil bubbles
souvenirs of beach walks
Thousand Island salad dressing
the book that made a difference
wind speed, measured at 33 feet above
ground by meteorologists
bar stools
studying with a great musician
an occulting light
Ming Dynasty art
sending flowers
finding a long-lost relative
sun visors
compact overnight bags
spot removers
cab services that show up on time
clouds pausing in their random, transient,
indifferent way
chariot races
the Triangle area of North Carolina
grabbing a pen
pizzaburgers for a hot lunch
good-humored patience

in painting, four colors making all colors

when anyone can look at the two of
  you and tell you are head over
  heels in love

Johnny Carson (comedian)

historical roadside markers

Hostess Sno Balls

the hanging ladder bars of a jungle gym

toggle clasps

tweezers getting the hair

not having to talk just to keep a
  conversation going

panda bears with white paws

left-handed boomerangs

lazily wiping your hands on your shirt

the pastiche of a colorful fishing village

terra firma

gestalt therapy

knowing that you own nothing but you
  have it all

taking a woodworking course

a rerun you haven't seen since childhood

going to bed early with a new mystery
  novel

today's special at a restaurant

carriage clocks

biking through the vineyards and stopping
  for a picnic

whispering in the dark

thinking of ways to deepen your knowledge

flying first-class for the first time
disaster movies
a Christmas card from a best friend
fishing lines
bringing a sense of adventure to a
    children's birthday party
a small-town library sale
dark clouds settling on the mountain ridges
asking a stranger where she got her
    handbag
a well-wishing attitude
something piquing your curiosity
homemade bookmarks
the art of paper-folding
refusing to let the snow stop you
the smell of a soothing bath salts
a typical arrangement or combination
    of words, collocations, such as "red
    apple" or "nice day"
the Heritage Trail of Indiana
admiring an old building
buying yourself flowers on Valentine's Day
secret herbs and spices in a recipe
a bison herd
a best-of-seven series
sheet music
changes that are reversible
shopping in factory outlet stores
the feeling of exhilaration when skiing
    down a slope really fast

summer dresses

the smartest thing you ever did

blue eyes

flip-flops in every conceivable color

dozing

parents crying from pride

tree swings

the origin of the hamburger: broiling hamburger patties with a thin slice of onion and placing them on a plate with home fries

knowing whose turn it is at a four-way stop

the Wright Brothers and Kitty Hawk, North Carolina

plain old bad habits

the angle at which light rays strike a surface and the angle at which they rebound from a surface

cross-country skiing through quiet forests

cabins with lobster traps stacked like cordwood in the backyard

having a foot in the stirrup

tying shirts up high

the natural randomness of drops of rain falling on grass

a party thrown in a big barn

the exciting moment when you first look out the window to see what the snow has done

a patient carpenter
Persian miniature paintings
using an ellipsis
cliffs like cathedrals and trees growing
    out of rocks
going to the same restaurant often enough
    to be given the same table
knowing how to do first aid
what you put ketchup on
retirement savings
tiny seashell "flowerpots" filled with wet
    sand, with little flowers stuck in
mischievous clouds with a fondness for
    popping out just as one decides to go
    in the ocean
puddle jumpers
bunches of drying herbs dangling from the
    rafters of a shady side porch
the jingle of a pet's ID tags
going to foreign movies
not underrating your own abilities
the joy of renunciation
railroad stations
laughing at soap operas
phrases like: to give someone the mitten,
    handbags at dawn
catching the romance of the moment
a good egg
rising earlier than the others, puttering
    softly, and quieting the beasts

a leisurely stroll bringing sensory
    delights
Christmas ornaments with inscribed dates
the panes of a greenhouse
the nubs, voids, and locks of a jigsaw
    puzzle
a baccalaureate
the pick of the litter
turkey cooked over a wood fire
falling asleep on someone's lap
the best dumb-luck things that ever
    happened to you
writing your spouse a love letter
the cadence of prayer on the first night
    of Hanukkah
summer mornings
The Art Institute, Chicago
"red carpet" welcomes
adventure sports
"Whatever you want, Mom!"
a new canvas
cash on hand
progressive relaxation: tightening and
    then loosening various muscles
lazily drifting on a raft, lying back and
    looking up
living in a charming town
getting carried away
being a little naughty
church choirs

eating over at someone's house
gathering a list of people's ideas of
cheap thrills
Midsummer Day
proms, gardenias, and moonlit dance halls
on the lake
loons yodeling
olive-colored duffel bags
sack races
a stroll on the lakeside footpath
the occasional screech of a gull
overhead
the sound a yawning dog emits when he
opens his mouth too wide
the beauty of flash memory
candlelight and Gregorian chants
"Row, Row, Row Your Boat" (song)
gouache, opaque watercolor
stretching to reach a parking lot's ticket
dispenser
corn relish
falling asleep to the sound of foghorns
Bill Nye the Science Guy
the back-and-forth dance of tennis players
accrued interest
playing all your iTunes songs, which
would take 1.6 days
memorizing the penal code
someone with boots on the wrong feet
cupcake papers

cabin fever

mock road signs as decorations

an almost full moon emerging from
behind the clouds

perfume oils

the pop songs that represent each decade
of your life

your favorite fictional character

farpotshket

the craziest thing you have done for love

sporting gear

bramble: raisins, cranberries in pastry,
topped with ice cream

Nubuck

nasturtiums climbing and tumbling with
bright flowers

hanging basket chairs

keeping the night-light on

dressing for pleasure

umpires' outfits

cookware racks

The Schoolhouse Shop, Chesterton,
Indiana

arms swinging while walking

the U.S. National Park Service

the places that don't change

reaching a compromise

knowing there are yoga poses for
everything, even unplugging your ears

Mickey Mouse

a tree old enough to shade most of a
    house
anything all spruced up
vanilla bread pudding with nutmeg
fruits to smell, such as early
    apples, fresh strawberries
travel games
those moments that go
    beyond words
a sofa ideal for vegging out and for chats
    with your legs curled up under you
trim on cars
beauty books
something best done alone, like eating all
    the pound cake right out of the box
an October owl in the dusk
getting one more item crammed into the
    garbage bag
a bonfire by an ice-skating rink
"Yes, dear."
positive psychology
pasta salad
deer slipping quietly across the lawn
    to eat the fallen apples
when you arrive at your destination just
    as a great song ends on the radio
an ornate building with gingerbread
    decoration
White Castle hamburgers
living in snow country

that over-the-rainbow feeling
fast food when you are craving it
engagement rings worn above
    wedding rings
when the audience smiles and taps
    their feet
white noise made from a blend of all
    audible frequencies
banded iron formations in Michigan
widening horizons, crisp nights, mild days
joining an Earthwatch expedition
the worm's-eye view
packing cookies in popped corn
a midlife adventure
going to the airport with a bag and
    passport and taking the first
    available flight
eating authentic hush puppies
    in Alabama
organizing your computer desktop
piglets and swine
the immense genius of Seurat, the pioneer
    of pointillism
bowling alleys
lying on your back in a snowy field,
    making an angel by moving your arms
    in arcs
chenille sweaters
plankton
kitchenettes in studio apartments

pure nonsense
old silent movies
the vocabulary of geology
winds, the unseen tides
"In today's job climate, you can't afford to
be a vanilla sundae. You need to be a
banana split." (Peter McCarthy)
visiting an apple farm
Treasure Island (book)
magazine-picture collages
intelligence and maturity
getting the guts to go jogging
the Swiss Alps
stiff collars
keeping notes on life
pelagic fish
a beautifully tiled bathroom
deciduous plants
window-shopping
the states you have visited
having a fireplace
no one in the steam room but you
the core curriculum
the joy of not cooking
coffee urns
misty mountain paths
a blueberry house with vanilla trim and
cranberry shutters
a child's wagon
a rolled lawn

complete disclosure
the midnight hungries
hiring a babysitter who's on a diet
editing a magazine or an article
quick turnaround time
golden retrievers
finding good reading material in someone
     else's bathroom
the ringmaster
doughnut glaze
facing the music
navy pants and light blue shirts
the clucking of a hen
hooks and eyes
a centerpiece of a container of colored
     pencils and a stash of paper
an aviator's scarf
uncharted seas
an extended vacation
PEZ candies
the setting sun's hallelujahs
a light touch
the smell of shampoo in your hair after
     a shower
chocolate raspberry truffle cake
being able to quit a bad job
routines for soothing the soul
ski-bobbing: riding downhill on a bicycle
     frame mounted on skis
wide-wale corduroy shirts

a snowfall of powdered sugar and a
     sprinkling of colored sugar crystals,
     white icing, and tiny candles
three bowls in Buddhist cooking: a large
     one for starch, a medium one for
     protein or grain, and a small one for
     beverage, salad, vegetable, or fruit
     dessert
throwing the windows open during a
     blizzard and enjoying the air
simple-hearted dreams of children
sheer sleeves in the glow of candlelight
process art
breakfast, the most important meal
snow outlining the elements of trees'
     architecture
eggplant Parmigiana
flowers poking out of crannied walls
vanilla-frosted, maple-frosted, and
     strawberry-frosted doughnuts
a field mouse scritch-scratching in the wall
a sentence you wish you had written
buying dinner and tickets to a hockey
     game
first buds
flo-thru tea bags
hiking the mesas looking for Anasazi
     caves and petroglyphs
a cat, out of boredom, starting to play
     with a toy

bad things that never happened or were
     not as bad as you feared
collecting baseball cards
an egg or omelet perfectly flipped
whole milk
catching the train just in time
yachts strung with Christmas lights
the romance of a Hallmark commercial
an architect of peace
the 19th-century engravings used in
     Merriam-Webster dictionaries
corsage pins
boosting your serotonin
dance studios
the many terms common to music and
     baseball
seedless raspberry jam
meeting someone at the airport
a swung half-door to the kitchen
hearing Santa and his reindeer on the roof
name-your-baby books
saddling a horse
getting to work five minutes early
shopping districts
the variety of lawn ornaments in your
     neighborhood
four hugs a day to fulfill "skin hunger"
alligators basking in the sun
multicolored anything
cinnamon coffeecake

perfect eyebrows
salty stories
over-35 basketball leagues
a body rejuvenated, spirit
    awake, and mind clear
steaming mugs of coffee
putting sprinkles on cupcakes
sweet insouciance
island air
writing a countermelody
couples moving closer and nuzzling
grade school
a tureen of hearty vegetable soup
the splash of a pool diver
inspiring yourself by self-encouragement
The Atlas of Experience by L. Van Swaaij
    and J. Klare
a sharp sense of the ironic
election night
tailoring learning to your life and interests
hiking to wildflower-spangled meadows
ceremonial peace pipes
proposing on bended knee
theater tickets for two
Rice Krispies cereal
cleaning rings with toothpaste
true madras: navy blue, maroon, mustard
    yellow—and it "bleeds"
not getting lost in a new town
zydeco dancing

teeter-totters

times to recall

cherries in your soda

sharing everything

leaves twinkling in the sunlight, spangling in the moonlight, dancing to the special music of raindrops on their thickness

the amusing shaking of a person's bottom while sharpening a pencil

lexicology

keeping a promise

pretending to take down an "important" phone message

freshman dorms

knowing the exceptions to grammar rules and the variants to spelling rules

adjustable pop-it beads

January in California

everyone jumping up and down at midnight to "Help Me, Rhonda" (song)

people knowing where they stand with you

homecoming mums

The Old Farmer's Almanac (book)

automatic transmission

West Side Story (movie)

strolling through a cool, dark pine forest

a mishmash

slow-churned ice cream
glasses that don't pinch your ears or nose
spooky sounds: tree branches scraping
a window; green wood in a house
structure, creaking and groaning;
roofs and walls expanding and
contracting; echoes, air traps; roof
shingles making the wind moan;
thumping water pipes
thinking twice before buying anything
the special symbols used by cartoonists to
replace swear words
a showery afternoon with great rolling
clouds
finding something you lost a long time ago
giving an affectionate nickname to
someone who doesn't have one
a Nantucket oil lamp
gymnasiums
the loose strand on each forkful of
spaghetti that beats you on the chin
cat-food packaging
modeling-agency models
sitting next to your best friend
beating your own drum
being apologetic
watching kids dive into a swimming pool
baseball diamonds
Beverly Hills' Rodeo Drive
business cards

the diner's 3 a.m. chili dogs and cheese
    fries

no loose ends

ultra-romantic dresses

using five free minutes to start an
    important project

a warm feeling of well-being

Australian wine

your favorite gadget

the richest of seasons

in winter, early snowdrops and autumn
    crocus under a bare orchard tree

slam dunks

gladiolus in acres of waving fields, in
    colorful floats in a parade, and fresh-
    cut in pretty bunches to take home

patio tables

estimating the temperature by counting
    the number of cricket chirps in 15
    seconds and adding 37

the cool breezes of a coastal summer day

the lead facial tissue that gets all the
    others going

ivory almond bark candy

a roaring fire scenting the air with wood
    smoke

the water cycle, the rock cycle, the carbon
    cycle, the nitrogen cycle

halcyon: calm, peaceful, happy, golden,
    prosperous, affluent

steak sauce and meat tenderizer
wild carnations
Coffee Pot Rapids, Idaho
conversations on paper
lumberjacks
rubber-soled deck shoes
a waterfront teahouse with a little
    footbridge
passion and compassion
really friendly TSA workers in their blue
    shirts
an acclaimed actor
"I love you."
chicken-filled tacos
bath sheets
restaurateurs
knowing—or being—that person who
    brightens a room just by entering it
a Crayola beginner's set
rechecking the mailbox to make sure your
    letter has gone down
catching an insect inside the house, and
    releasing it outside
learning a great synonym
the guts to "go for it"
nylon
floats and fireworks
a toast to the bride
a mini kick in the pants in the right
    direction

pedal-boating in Bermuda
battery testers
cloisonné, the art of blending fired enamel
    and brass
calligraphied expressions
lowered voices
a gaggle of geese
precooked bacon
going sockless
the names of the sizes of hailstones
cooking on a gas stove
an old railroad station
assistance dogs
green lawns shaded by willows and
    carpeted with daffodils
gingerbread-flavored memories of
    childhood
when you build a fire outside and it pops
ancient Rome's aqueduct system
someone who thinks you are hot
cuddling up to your lover for warmth
Chinese New Year
sharing all the awesome little things that
    happen during the day
bathing beaches
close-up photographic techniques
Show and Tell, followed by a good nap
when a recipe surpasses your
    expectations
a lick and a promise

rough-and-tumble clothes
pushing your luck
the fat-over-lean rule in oil painting and
	pastel
having a childhood playhouse
new stanzas to the poems written on the
	hillside, meadow, and riverbank
stretching marshmallows like taffy
jasmine flower
trying out for cheerleading
stately homes
leaving fresh cookies for Santa
buying hardcover books
retiring in New Zealand
reveling in time alone
a realistic home budget
testing a "wet paint" sign for yourself
white place cards
pets in line for the fire hydrant
being happy sharing quiet moments
surf fishing
rearranging the garage so that your band
	can practice in it
picking out a card and sending it to
	someone who would never expect it
precariously tall lemon meringue
tracking your time to see how you use it
appreciating the old, slower methods,
	like math on paper instead of with
	a calculator

ice-cream makers
a date on Saturday night
that happy-go-lucky feeling
seeing your breath exhaled as a frosty
    puff
the creak of an old door or gate
tiny deep-fat fryers
clearing the table after a meal
turning telephone ringers off
updating clothes
listening to the wind
cubbyholes
a new fact you recently learned
traveling your own road
the collective unconscious
not despising what you cannot get
admirable fortitude
a carriage ride in Acadia National Park
"honest and simple," the highest
    compliment you can pay
furniture that has personality
letting fireworks send chills up your spine
dogs that hold their leashes in their
    mouths
"Way to go!"
having a good poker face
birds on electric wires not getting
    electrocuted because they don't
    complete a circuit or create a short
    because they are not grounded

broiled cheeseburgers

teaching grammar in a way a child
     understands

a raccoon peering out through his
     permanent sunglasses

balloon racing

birthdays, anniversaries, and red-letter
     days

turquoise umbrellas shading white
     ironwork tables and chairs

the organization of your life

returning a smile

raisin racks for drying California grapes

minerals that color stone formations
     deep black and red, purple, green,
     and orange

ripe peaches on a summer's eve

New Jersey: crossroads of the Revolution,
     Miss America, wild orchids, pixie
     moss, Atlantic City

pencils, pens, a sketchbook, books to
     help identify wildflowers or birds,
     and maps

men who wear glasses

"bats in the belfry"

the center of a cinnamon bun

collections from everyday life

a writer with an idea

an easy place to tie your shoes

racing a bike

getting to appear on *The Tonight Show*

your first dorm room

merging traffic

the cat acting foolish

knowledge of arcane whys and hows

winning on a technicality

multiplying sunlight with mirrors

sensuous scents

cattle placidly munching their way through the meadows

climbing a tree to do some constructive daydreaming

old boats' quiet, graceful sails

breakfast cooked over an outdoor fire

safety valves

people who have it all together

arriving home from the bookshop or the library with an armload of volumes begging to be read

orange and lime sherbets

the three-second attention span of a goldfish

listening to the beat of music and doing nothing, just listening to the drums

nonchalance

shaking a sugar packet vigorously to move the contents to the bottom before tearing it open

baby cereal

your favorite new TV shows

when a suede purse's color does
    not rub off on your clothes
your own office
someone laughing in his or
    her sleep
the expressive faces of pansies
building a dollhouse
fellow airline passengers
skipping among the waves and diving
    beneath the swells
the return of curls, ponytails, crew cuts
wide-open floor space
learning about Indo-European languages
a new theater multiplex
a bobbing Adam's apple
practice runs visualized
flower petals tossed instead of rice at a
    wedding
turning off the lamp when the sun makes
    it unnecessary
trying to work things out on your own
remembering when kids used to want to
    be President
a motorized tie rack
working independently
blueberry pails
dwelling in possibility
seeing a blimp land
eating Oreo cookies and then looking at
    your teeth

relative humidity

taking a short stroll before deciding on
new shoes

preparing for tomorrow

singing to iTunes and looking up lyrics
online as the song plays

The Middle (TV show) on ABC using this
book as a prop in numerous episodes

the aroma of basil

time-lapse photography of a thunderstorm

country auctions

feeling heady with optimism and warmth

panning for gold

camping when the weather was great, the
kids had a ball, nature was at it best,
the family reconnected, and there
was no electricity involved

shell mobiles

automobile racing

learning 100 basic words in sign language

a table covered with glue sticks, glitter,
pipe cleaners, googly eyes

the slowed sounds of an Austrian zither

making sure all your friends get home
safely from holiday parties

when the exact amount you want to tip
rounds up to a bill you have in your
wallet

what's stored in your closets

succulence

lukewarm water

inexpensive cafeteria lunches

finding out that for years you've
mispronounced one of your favorite
words

learning-to-write-cursive pens

cheating death

spotting bobolinks and short-billed marsh
wrens

the excitement of a storm and the sudden
transformation of the landscape

the Na Pali Coast of Kauai

creating your own sunshine

finding the quiet "center" of your life your
own way

Gatorade kegs

burnt butter, brown sugar cupcakes

goodnights

"It is by studying little things that we
attain the great art of having as little
misery and as much happiness as
possible." (Samuel Johnson)

fresh formats

throwing eggs or water balloons to people
in a contest

harbor houses

accomplishing what you undertake

sniffing the air to see whether snow is
coming

Easter breads

thinking happy summer thoughts

the county seat

setting up a breakfast tray the night before

a carpet rake

the small metal ring on a ballpoint
pen that separates the top
half from the bottom half

making a great cup of coffee

play being a rest from the world

kames, kettles, and eskers formed
by glaciers

the perfect outdoor café where you can
hang out with a newspaper, sip,
nibble, people-watch

lightly battered fried zucchini blossoms

an apple and a candy bar in your
Christmas stocking

a T-bone, served for two

you-had-to-be-there moments

touching wood

dust on the goldenrod

clairvoyance

waterfront properties in Maine

a place where small kittens sit sunning
themselves on stone walls

manners being the happy ways of doing
things

palm reading

harmless impulsiveness

Watermelon Day at camp or the park

Adam's Peak in Sri Lanka, with a hollow
    at the top venerated as the footprint
    of Buddha, Adam, and Shiva
dinner rolls
white chocolate
hockey boards
when people say nice things behind your
    back
handing out paychecks
struggling with a decision, then knowing
    in your heart you made the right one
summer squash on a sunny yellow
    tablecloth
picking flowers here and there, then
    putting them between the pages of
    a big heavy book to dry
waiting for a chance to say something
solar panels soaking up the sun
taking a meal in the fresh air and sunshine
canals with sluice gates
Rockefeller Center, New York City
Indonesia's 17,508 islands
"When things get tough, the tough get
    going."
articulating passion
quiet libraries
making a horse gallop
board game nights
a theatrical streak
glasses you only wear at home

writing with chalk on the driveway

spotting typos before something is sent

shaving a peach

your body temperature reaching its lowest
point around 4 a.m. and then rising
again and, when it does, you begin to
wake up

the smells of pine and fresh coffee

mini-meals

iced tea loaded with slices of lemon, lime,
and oranges

that first leap into a pool even though you
know it is going to be cold

a June bride

taking a complete rest

corn shocks tepeed in the fields

the tiny depressions on an English muffin

the Florida Keys

your home's resident squirrel, who
sits next to the trunk of a tree
and nibbles nuts loudly

cayenne pepper

cock-a-doodle-do

wind-whistling days of January

buying yourself a toy you wanted as a child

blue-and-white chintz

starting to make things happen

1954

someone who switches the laundry
for you

overnight trips

walking with erect carriage, a step springy
   and elastic

Braille markings on drive-up ATMs

a weathered boardwalk

concentrating on being you

cotton balls

blow dryers

sunrise at 5 a.m.

stonewashed jeans

the first guess always being the best on
   a multiple-choice question

inn rooms equipped with terry-cloth robes

cheeks tingling in the winter

alternating between reading a novel and
   looking at the hilltop skyline

penny loafers with the pennies stuck in
the parts of Wisconsin
   that are east of Florida

repositioning the Christmas
   tree lights so no two of
   the same color are together

D-Day

getting kids to do the activity for which
   they have the longest attention span

sewing all your loose buttons on

bones for dogs

laughing at someone's favorite story—again

catching a Hail Mary pass

christenings

going birding
driving defensively
a stitch in time
the discreet murmur of voices
The People's Almanac (book series)
a brood of chicks, hens
the slight trace of criminality one feels
    when having a lover's keys duplicated
turning a house into a home
dressing up
successful "quality assurance"
rededicating your life to something more
    meaningful
the smell of flowers through the screens
stretching your limbs like a starfish
the Mississippi River
taking something under advisement
the monuments in Washington, D.C., lit up
    at night
starting a pogo stick fad
the fast-falling November twilight
"Hey, hey, we're the Monkees, and people
    say we monkey around. But we're too
    busy singing to put anybody down."
    (theme song from the TV show)
body language
FUBAR: Fouled Up Beyond All
    Recognition
ceramic beads
how-to books

snacks after a movie

transits into vanished or imaginary worlds

a journal accepting all that you write with
no judgments

chopping wood

a cute plaid dress

scheduling appointments

getting a whiff of that first ocean breeze

jalapeño peppers

checkmarks in book margins for parts you
think are important

quantum theory

electric trains

thatched-roof cottages

a watchmaker tilting tiny cogs and wheels
into place

a good salad spinner

cakes of soap

the candymaker's art

dark blue sky

Burger King Whoppers

a plenteous supply of picnic food

giving the perfect gift: a private reflection
about someone, and a deep desire to
please him or her

a boxed set you've been wanting and can
afford

not checking email on vacation

adequate preparation

playing freeze-tag in the sprinkler

sandwiches called Tex-Mex, smørrebrød,
    muffuletta
falling asleep on the couch
a beautiful old book crammed with
    scraps of past and present pleasures:
    postcards, fabric samples, dried
    flowers
sitting outside for an hour each day, when
    possible
rubber rafts
popping Goldfish crackers
muffins as big as softballs
traffic lights
turrets and towers
knowing the difference between Jekyll
    and Hyde
peanut butter so sticky you could mortar
    bricks with it
classical music
collecting things for a future home
tintypes of grandparents in silver frames
standing next to someone you love
a wandering artist's journal
free-range chicken raising
scenes from old movies
an epiphany
box offices
classy uniforms
washing the car mats
Harry Connick Jr.'s music

drinking hot drinks through a straw so
    you don't burn your mouth
when someone tells you that you have
    something in your teeth
a warmer-than-normal winter after a slew
    of very cold ones
today's promise becoming tomorrow's joy
holding a jujube up to the cinema screen
    in order to determine its color
picking strawberries or tomatoes
each footstep, a unique event in itself
hutches, highboys, and buffet tables
raking a big pile of leaves and jumping in
choreographers magnifying, exaggerating,
    and beautifying how people move
orchards heavy with blushing red apples
    and flocks of turkeys being fattened
    for the approaching holiday feasts
apothecary jars
things falling into place
snow-capped volcanoes
software engineering
recreation and leisure
varicolored beauty in an old-fashioned
    garden
your first love letter
the shy/proud look of children receiving
    awards
prismed crystal chandeliers
a red canoe

on a train, experiencing a journey of
    endless surprises
the Lascaux cave paintings
fraternity softball games
indentations that appear in carpets after a
    piece of furniture has been moved
learning how to polka
shredding and recycling office paper
the art of rowing
careful use of a staple gun
remembering the year a song came out
nacho cheese from a pump
subtle color gradations
stories of famous scientists who inspire
    you
dear hearts and gentle people
spending a day when you take
    cabs everywhere or walk
    everywhere
mouthwash that works but
    is not harmful
pregnant women
casting a wide net
Madison Square Garden
booths in park bench style
times when showing off is okay
snow crunching underfoot, snug in its
    snowsuit and boots
cackles in a henhouse
the enthusiasm of an entrepreneur

white sales
the spirit of the American
when you hear someone smile over the
    phone
the hustle of go-getters
the seascapes of southern Rhode Island
a beautiful, old, renovated mill
spontaneity
The Good Housekeeping Cookbook
silly songs in the car
sundresses and pinafores you can layer
    over T-shirts
garden hoses
the game Categories—listing diseases
    beginning with *L*, puddings beginning
    with *W*
kitty litter that stays in the box
oodles of noodles
closing your eyes and breathing in
cotton tunics
home brews
snow croquet
authentic Mexican food
going back to square one
seasonal beverages during the holidays
erect posture
seaweed tapestries woven with shells, fish
    bones, feathers, sponge bits
Ripley's Believe It or Not
someone being your every dream

U-shaped desks
porcupines scratching
a trail of thin mist rising along the
    whispering brook
the moment while exercising when
    thought fades away
American fries, thick potato chips
jazz dances
house cats in a sparring match
little brass pitchers
a large tree with an umbrella of 25 feet
a sheltering frieze framing the sky
secret agents
pricing items for a garage sale
watching people interact
an in-the-water boat show
intricate colored chalk drawings on the
    sidewalk
the smell of rainstorms and roses and
    fresh-cut grass
three-ring binders
silent prayer
sitting in bed watching the sun rise over
    the park
the giant fireplaces of a castle
cats: Abyssinian, alley, Angora, Burmese,
    calico, Cheshire, domestic shorthair,
    Himalayan, Manx, Persian, seal point,
    Siamese, tiger, tortoiseshell
reams of paper

fish sticks and homemade tartar sauce
taking your time
being soothed like a baby
the college reunions you attend
baseball lights coming on
people who hold the elevator doors so
    they don't close in your face
swell sounds
food debris under a high chair following
    an attempted feeding
careful speech
promenading
no-bake pies
maximizing the positive things
clicking castanets
a cat that sleeps on a pad on your office
    desk while you work all day
a Christmas tree decorated in tiny
    flickering white lights and gingham
    bows
when Mr. Right trips over your beach
    blanket
coffee carts loose in the building
piney woods
tandoori chicken and mango lassi
the difference between realistic and
    stupid campaign promises
your tummy wanting something yummy
flitting around for pleasure in
    the evening

having no TV or telephone or radio or
    Wi-Fi in the inn room
September in the country
*The Baby Blue Cat and the Dirty Dog
    Brothers* (Ainslie Pryor)
watching a cook prepare luncheon while
    sitting on the lawn with a view of the
    marina
attending a yacht race
designing a photo calendar
the Tour de France bicycle race
calling friends
rosy cherub cheeks
"Mum's the word."
goals written in sand
happy unplanned moments
someone with a "force field"
airing the quilts, thinking about the
    gardens, taking off the storm
    windows, going for long walks,
    buying a new hat
boudoir stools
buckets of golf balls
TV studios
slow-cooked oatmeal
bluish-gray Australian cattle dogs
unity
balls-out fun
a stickler for details
being on the edge of one's seat

songs that never lose their appeal

track lighting

walking in the opposite direction from
someone on a foggy day and watching
the other person disappear

colors against a good tan

a baby's ring

fruit or vegetable pictures for the kitchen

uncrowded places to shop

white dress shirts with black trousers

Cheshire cats

country hutches

plate-spinning acrobatics

something more powerful, universal,
peaceful

a chili cook-off in March

traveling with many maps folded into the
glove compartment of memory

salted caramel frosting

madeleines, little French sponge cakes in
the shape of scallop shells

riding the crest of a wave

a wedding you attend, giving you a chance
to reflect back on your wedding day
and feel renewed love for each other

Florida: whitewashed hotels, sponges,
alligators, glass-bottomed boats

teatime meringues, sweet and lightweight

a box that slides neatly into an exact
space

a cherry-vanilla milkshake and a Brazier
burger
the relief of being unpacked after a move
sails against blue water
"You are never too old to set another
goal or to dream a new dream."
(C.S. Lewis)
the shortest day of the year
stowing away memories of wonderful
moments
posters from the 1960s and 1970s that you
had in your room, dorm room, first
apartment
yellow: banana squashes, corn, peppers,
sweet potatoes, bananas, lemons,
grapefruit, pineapple
believing in one great love
tempura dishes
I Spy (TV show)
the 1610 population of the American
colonies: 350
advances in science and technology
the zigzag ridges on the top of a brown
paper bag
candles at the windows
marine biology
fiber optics
the excited sounds of foosball
Telegraph Hill in San Francisco
back scrubbers

stone bridges
watching gardens and children grow
fall visitors
common courtesy
extra sweaters, boots, parkas for winter
sterling-silver tips for the collar of a
    Western shirt
making a lifestyle change
dining out
animals taking their time, not rushed like
    humans
origins of words
horseradish sneaking up on you
an irresistible, untimely urge to dance
using a kite as a wall hanging
hospice workers
the ride being worth the trouble
Hungarian goulash
striking gold
playing while someone mows the lawn
heavy pots
public-address systems
apple orchards wearing their first
    red blush of harvest
designing a race car
the head on a freshly made egg cream
petting a seal or other animal at the zoo
dreaming the impossible dream
branches of trees silvered with crystal or
    flocked with snow

tea bag tags
Norway, Land of the Midnight Sun
bright buttons
the red wedding dress of Chinese brides
the extra car keys
old clothes
the house wren's exuberant trill
knowing what can happen in a second
small dinner parties
fusilli
Flanders, Connecticut
drop waists
a stack of buttered toast
direct perception, a different kind of
    seeing, that is an integral part of the
    thinking and creative process
variegated garden flowers such as
    carnations and tulips
snatched sidewalk kisses
bargains galore
spending two days in an Inuit village
    above the Arctic Circle
sorority or fraternity memories
the breath you take before signing your
    name on a loan or lease
staying out of the rat race
brass horns
love under an umbrella
the things we haven't been taught being
    the things we know best

the 64 squares on a chess or checkers
    board
the most perfect of any music filling
    the air
worn brick paths with moss-filled cracks
"Better ask twice than lose your way
    once." (Danish proverb)
a billboard that makes you think
    or laugh
rhinestone buttons
the "law of threes"
a cedar-paneled stateroom
nonpolluting fuel like hydrogen fuel cells
ideas falling into place
making a connecting flight with plenty
    of time to go to the bathroom, call
    home, and pick up a magazine and
    something to drink
wassail, a punch made of cider, lemonade,
    orange juice, brown sugar, spices, and
    baked apples, served in a large bowl
things turning out best for the people
    who make the best of the way things
    turn out
rags of white clouds rolling in from
    the sea
astronomers observing
weeds that are prettier than the grass they
    spring up in
Gossip Girl (TV show)

testing a few phrases of a remembered
    song
bread stuffing
saying what's on your mind
finding out the test or quiz is shorter than
    expected
mini hamburgers/sliders by the bagful
being happy
knowing what you do best, then doing it
beef jerky at the cash register
a race on the beach
heartwarming news
Russian hats
meeting people at parties
camera bags
scruffy skiers
opening milk cartons
botanical photographs and watercolors
Great Barrington, Massachusetts
colorful computer-generated schematics
    manipulated in three-dimensional
    space
watching the monitor as your blood
    pressure is being taken
the courthouse square
neighborhood shops
stirring up the dust in your room while the
    sun shines through a hole in the curtain
solidus, the slanted line between words
immaculate lawns

floating on your back in the pool
an overnight at a nice hotel in the city
hope chests
turning the corner of your own street
a staircase of huge boulders
a catchy theme song for a TV show
the sedatives of wood smoke and
    candlelight
paper airplane flying
Mount Baldy, Indiana Dunes: a living dune,
    moving southward about 4 feet a year
discovering your own quiet joy
a ranch-style wrought-iron triangle for
    announcing dinner
knit ribbing on cuffs
getting a stuck basketball out by using
    another ball
the secret hideout of your youth
velvet voices
an old-fashioned flavor and honest
    function in a room
Black Forest ham
Perrier-shaped glassware
hot-sun yellows
using part of your lunch hour for spiritual
    renewal
judging a bakery on the quality of its fresh
    bread
candle-lighting, turkey-stuffing, mistletoe-
    hanging

sunset over a harbor

drinking from the garden hose

something happening by chance and
turning out well

a scrawny pup with a high-frequency tail

using gift cards or rewards certificates so
something costs almost nothing

mullioned windows

pets whose names match their look/color
or personality

comfortable armchairs

"Once upon a time . . ."

wearing something brilliant and watching
other people's reactions

warmth when you need it

the type of song performed by Venetian
gondoliers

trapdoors

soft pretzels with grains of hard, coarse
salt, served with sunny yellow mustard

finding the perfect illustrator for your book

ranch life

sitting around the dining room table after
dinner and enjoying long conversations

gulls diving for quarry along the Atlantic

tie-dyed rainbow clothing

the little red wagon under the Christmas
tree

unendangered species

dipping your toes in a fountain

an old-fashioned herb bed
a late breakfast
Leve fit quod bene fertur onus, "That load
  becomes light which is cheerfully
  borne."
landscapers' pickup trucks
when there was a floppy disk drive
knowing which wines pair with foods
kayak races
a bottle opener/knife/corkscrew
  combination
doing your own thing
a square deal
sitting on a porch or bench reading
  a print newspaper
choosing a neighborhood
ducks fishing for their dinners
fairy lights
rummage sales
"hanging out" and remembering
  why you like each other
baking powder
a book bag with large ring binder
  (different section for each subject),
  Glamour magazine, Sharpies in five
  colors, a travel pack of Kleenex,
  hairbrush, *Elements of Style*
sidewalk tables
a student about to receive his/her degree
Himalayan snowfields

moneyed enclaves turning into relaxed
seaside towns, mansions giving way
to clam shacks, kayaks outnumbering
yachts
new wallpaper
the dog head-tilting at you
escape artists
beating a personal record
freshly cracked black pepper in spaghetti
carbonara
your game face
the trumpet of a train passing
what you thought sushi would taste like
before you ever tried it
the ping-pong of batted tennis balls
magic shows
discovering an etymology
making up dreams in bed
phrases from Shakespeare: rotten apple,
a man of few words, cold comfort,
mind's eye, one fell swoop, neither
here nor there, it's Greek to me, it's a
mad world, haven't slept a wink, seen
better days
meringue pies: foam-white clouds gilded
with caramelized froth
a pond that changes color in different
shades of light
scratched-stucco farmhouses
working with a personal trainer

John Muir, America's first heroic
    preservationist
tree branches playing tag
time cards
having to wander through a maze of ropes
    at an airport or bank even when
    you're the only person in line
the shopping list on the fridge
thinking someone is terrific
cleanliness
the rich, deep purples of late August
translucent hair color with subtle shadings
fossilized dinosaur tracks
hula-hooping
a word you overuse
an opportunity to use the diamond lane
palm-fringed beach
mixing real flowers and silk leaves
farm-fresh food
wanting to gain some perspective on
    your life, finding answers to unsolved
    dilemmas, and contemplating future
    directions
TUMS antacid
the cardboard snowflake you made when
    you were little
last light
a much-needed afternoon nap
confectioners' sugar
forthcoming attractions

baseballs signed by famous players
the Borscht Belt
being great company
a commemorative stamp series
101 Dalmatians (story)
pruning trees
patio dining in summer
Icelandic ponies
"My Girl" (song)
quitting your day job
going online and answering someone's
    question
shadows cast by shutters against shiny
    white walls
mood lighting
smoothtop stoves
the chatter of a group of women
a pretty face
the large hearts of heroes
organizing office yoga sessions
food straight from your grocer's freezer
vicarious savoring
a marriage proposal hidden in the solution
    to a crossword puzzle
tiered jewelry boxes
being dapper at home
glass slippers
a refill without asking
Mel Brooks's *Blazing Saddles, High
    Anxiety, Young Frankenstein* (movies)

the tininess of kids' underwear and socks
melting snow making streams along the
roadside
one-act plays
going tramping, getting outdoors and
basking, or just gloating and being
content
campfire parties in the desert
drink-of-water requests at bedtime
downtime to reset the mind's clock
taking a flying leap
keeping takeout food warm while you
drive home
seedlings opening paired leaflets on
the windowsill
rebuilding an engine
hands-free toilet bowl cleaner
wide-brim hats with black velvet–ribbon
trim
pebbled streets
the benefits of getting older
being realistic
the tractor on the farm
a dog that stops barking
medieval houses
the Metropolitan Museum of Art's
Christmas tree
learn-a-language playing cards
pumpkin, zucchini, and cranberry breads
rolling the rugs back for dancing

gaping at wacky Americana on Route 66
butterflies gathering in bunches in the air
taking the extra minute to notice
remaining calm when you find out you
    need glasses
a blaze of color
an optimistic forecast
mail holding and forwarding
an island frothed with wildflowers
lots of books to read in case the weather
    changes your plans
taking care
a chauffeur in uniform
honey-warm fall days
sliced oranges
little feet in the sand
a vow of silence
at water's edge, empty shells that whisper
    when summer waves turn them
"Half a loaf is better than none."
reviving an old plan
a full paper tray in the copier
a hardware store on a Saturday
ankle-tickling sleepwear
throwing out the towel at wrestling meets
Steve Jobs, entrepreneur
a half-moon-shaped desk like Noah
    Webster's
watch caps with rolled-up brims
seeing fjords from an icebreaker

appurtenances
Weight Watchers
spicy-hot enchiladas
how much better a salad can be at a
    restaurant
pocket watches
successfully giving someone directions in
    your town
knowing you're absolutely unique
lobster mac and cheese
the political convention weeks
the inertia that overcomes drivers when
    they see police on the road
red carnations with green candles
Steve Martin, comedian
mountain biking
doing tai chi outdoors
wadded-up pieces of paper
gallons, bushels, pecks
low, rolling thunder in late fall
the faint aroma of anchovy emanating
    from Worcestershire sauce
funny T-shirts for kids like, "I'm 4 years
    old and there's nothing you can do
    about it"
hypoallergenic blankets
menus from country inns
a citrine ring
taking lots of notes
open-air beauty

full-service gas stations
beech leaves delicate as a fluff of silk
the first time you felt your baby kicking
design elements: shape, size, color,
     texture, line, direction, value
chanting singsong lessons in a one-room
     schoolhouse
a stool at the soda fountain of an old
     drugstore
New York strip sirloin, cut extra thick
rainy days
working at the polls
minding your own business
the warming of the heart
morning weather reports
the real-life places behind your desktop
     backgrounds
governor's palace lights
fresh-laid eggs
the realities of marriage
untangling dogs from leashes
pub food
dreams and imagination
times when you are not motivated to do
     anything at all
enjoying morning coffee on the terrace of
     your hotel room
the summer song of mowers
coonskin caps
round barns

James Jeans's theory of molecules
  scattered in the atmosphere, that
  chances are we each have five
  molecules from the last breath of
  Julius Caesar
inventing a new dance
eating popcorn and cracking nuts
saving mementos
Scottish tam-o'-shanters
violent, paralyzing snowstorms—
  midweek
waffle houses
Welcome Wagon
paper cups with pullout handles
China-red satin pajamas
languages escaping their countries of
  origin
being known for one sensational recipe
the place where one sock in every laundry
  load disappears to
entering a zone or the flow of creativity
yachting blazers
four-leaf clovers
a baby's first solid food
10 minutes used wisely
soaking a pan before trying to clean it
anyone who pushes in his or her chair
  when he or she gets up from the table
white lies
rear-window defoggers

your-weight-and-fortune machines
context clues
cruise ships
bad-weather get-togethers
Maypo oatmeal
the best fruit market
a puppy at the gnaw-it-all stage
a light-drenched family room
the romance potential of a vacation
the opportunity to thank your
    lucky stars
dealing cards for a game of solitaire
the midnight sun in Reykjavik, Iceland
eating off glass plates
unusually large things like an 800-pound
    pumpkin or 6-foot-long pencil
the roar and crackle of a log fire's
    beginnings and the whispering
    snicker of its slow dying
Tennessee: Nashville, marble, green,
    horses, Grand Ole Opry
carrying 10 books home from the library
hearing church bells
the firewall of your computer
yellow Goldenrod writing tablets
mango fried rice
the sloping floor of a movie house
the songs of summer slowly revealed
a small-town Main Street filled with
    tony shops

Stratton, Stowe, and Mad River Glen in
    Vermont; Sugarloaf in Maine
days for special projects you've been
    procrastinating about
noted artists
hoping or praying something will work
    out
the muscles of athletes' legs
a boule of sourdough
a couch you can stretch out on
architecture: inhabited sculpture
log rollers
two-piece tank swimsuits
writing down a significant memory from
    each year of your life
the silence and big logo before a film
boat shoes in navy blue
getting permanent marker off a dry-erase
    board
hasty pudding
brooms and mops
learning new things
discovering a great secret
birthstone rings
dormant volcanoes
the parts of your job that you love
hot cross buns on Easter morning
a puppy or kitten's sideways run
snare drums
a full-fledged home-cooked dinner

art for the hell of it

snuggling into a soft chair with
a good book

fireside log lighters

the renowned Inn at Little Washington

sunflower ranches and farms

looking at the western sky in mid-evening

beveled mirrors

driving the kids to school in bad weather
or when special projects are being
transported

the way baby spider plants hang from the
mother plant

your quirky tastes

a cordless immersion blender

word nerds

perfecting a tennis serve

the few seconds of pleasure before the
aftertaste of a diet drink sets in

wedding rings

Norman Rockwell's *Stockbridge at
Christmas* painting

"Never complain, never explain."

railroads adopting the foolproof red,
yellow, green system and traffic
engineers later borrowing this for
stoplights

a porkpie hassock with a knob on top

when cicadas stop making noise

teaching one another

wearing cowboy boots east of the
    Mississippi River
popping corn
angle parking
a tavern table
knowing the freshest items are at the
    back of the grocer's shelf
iridescence
measuring flour
rows of mailboxes hungrily awaiting their
    daily feeding
playing hide-and-seek in the park
a waiter presenting a spoken menu
rugby shirts
cocker spaniels
personalizing a jar of spaghetti sauce
volunteer tutors
the weaving of Triscuits
Valentine, Texas and Nebraska
chives, bergamot, sweet cicely, purslane,
    pennyroyal, betony, mallow, dill,
    coriander, saffron, anise, borage,
    caraway, marigold, violet, bog myrtle,
    clary sage, soapwort, meadowsweet,
    rose, and lemon verbena
using a brightly colored quilt for a
    tablecloth
a very slight digression
small, moist, bite-size muffins served
    slightly warm

a beautiful fountain in the town center
park

an *ebelskiver* pan for making puffy,
sphere-shaped Scandinavian
pancakes with jam or fruit inside

wonderful tiny restaurants in old houses
with slanted floors

Mazda Miatas

Stars Hollow, Connecticut, the setting of
Gilmore Girls (TV show)

the worm, the spiral part of corkscrew

a scene that is highly paintable and
photographable

learning to do self-hypnosis

unforgettable friends

a small sheepskin rug

being 72.8 percent water

a baby's first tooth

clocks that tick

being sensuous

wanting your teddy bear

silver doilies

cloud-high trees

barbershop quartet contests

ad hoc: for a specific purpose
or special case

great walkable cities

Washington's famous crossing of the
Delaware

brushing your son's hair

the sound of sneakers squeaking against
the floor during basketball games
hot, moist washcloths in some restaurants
and airplanes
Sesame Street (TV show)
snails sleeping for years without eating
breaking in a new hat
a Sharpie when you need one
mnemonic devices
porch swings
the tang of autumn fires
Harry Potter and Lemony Snicket
the shadows of the clouds passing over
the Earth
research fellowships
"not for all the tea in China"
exiting a museum via the gift shop
oxymorons: jumbo shrimp, pretty ugly,
holy war, plastic glass, artificial grass
planets and their moons
airy netting
quotations you want to think about
a nice roommate to help with the rent
dinner-on-the-farm restaurants
a shish kebab of herbs on charred meat,
alternated with slices of blackened
onion
crafts to make, puzzles to solve, tricks to
do, experiments to perform; things to
build, cut out, color, cook, and grow

water's shiny surface
the old college try
fabric-protector sprays
places where you can lunch in a swimsuit
muscle memory
a bright green parrot
spinning around on a diner stool
casement windows
unusual decorating finds
cultured gray or pink pearls
Tribune Tower, Chicago
Dr. Seuss never defining
    the words he made up
never being discouraged
things that fascinated you as a child
when you start thinking about where
    you'll take your vacation
shirtsleeves
a friend running in a marathon
Army-Navy stores
the season of the harvest moon
lace-thin johnnycakes with butter and
    syrup
eleven square miles of paradise: Block
    Island
wine country
starting a new knitting project
that there is no butter in buttermilk, egg in
    eggplant, pine or apple in pineapple,
    or ham in hamburger

twice-baked potatoes

streaming the movie you want to watch

throwing a 30-yard pass

dancing to music coming from your
headphones

computer nerds with a large collection of
pens in their shirt pockets

X-Acto knives

ancient gray stones and white picket
fences

watching TV with a bowl of ice and
a fan

breathing deeply

the abundant hillsides of Burgundy

American English

visiting the lobster tank at the grocery
store

night coming in like a black silk cloak,
silently folding itself around us

that the summit of Mount Everest is
marine sandstone

24-hour stores

dentists who don't expect you to carry
on a conversation with a mouthful
of novocaine and their fingers in
your mouth

unbitten fingernails

picking a passion flower

toaster waffles

commending a colleague

someone who is magnetic in a quiet
sense and equanimous in disturbing
situations
the shadows of deep water
the visible spectrum of light
your car radio's presets
boxwood hedges
designer pizzas
a flip book from one haircut to the next,
made of photos, so you can watch
your hair grow
Traverse City, Michigan
faking your way through unintelligible
lyrics
loving fresh bread
visiting museums
rope tricks
vanilla-colored beaches
being happily alone in a crowd
"Indian Summer" by Emily Dickinson
Stradivarius violins
traveling first class on a train
the kitchen
humble abodes
eating at the bar in a favorite restaurant
spinach salad
getting less wet walking in the rain and
least wet standing still
Crate and Barrel stores
sweet dreams

packing a picnic and taking your family
    on a trip to the country
pulling out some old favorite games:
    Monopoly, Clue, Parcheesi
Reader's Digest word quizzes
calligraphy pens
spring bringing out the motorcyclists
being a pumpkin, a skeleton, an astronaut,
    or a bumblebee for Halloween
straight-backed chairs for working
an English pub in the Berkshires
stereoscopic photographs
    and a special viewer
a black suit
pencil boxes
draping a night table with fabric
writers needing solitude as others
    need sleep
taking lots of microbreaks
waxed paper
snapping the lock on the swimming pool
    fence for the last time
verbal sunshine
Peoria farm equipment
sending Christmas cards
the far corners of the Earth
playpen toys
painting the front door a bright color and
    adding a brass knocker
tufted cushions

a weekly email newsletter you love receiving

the widening and lengthening of flower petals

western forests

cats exploring in bushes and walking along the tops of low garden walls

your favorite face

priming a kitchen pump to draw a glass of clear, cold well water

when it's business, not personal

newly discovered chemical elements

being immersed in dramatic mountain scenery

two-handed solitaire

the swinging of the pendulum

solacing others

horns of plenty

recognizing the obvious

the hiss of a heavy rain

"Looney Tunes" cartoons

rustic-look furniture

people who make you listen to an entire song or comedy routine before you get the beep on their answering machine

meditation downloads

museum shops and bookstores for a quiet browse

round Band-Aids

serene, sun-splashed scenes
becoming friends with the other person
at the event who does not know
anyone there
a cabin by the side of a huge northern lake
thin-handled modern silverware
beef chop suey
stainless-steel cookware
split-collar sweaters
a line of poetry that keeps cycling through
your mind
big country dining rooms
skinny breadsticks
diligence and industry
prandial (cooking) skills
a sailboat passing within 50 yards of
where you're sunning yourself
fireworks effects: Chrysanthemum,
Weeping Willow, Battle in the Clouds
a ball hit in the center of the fairway
doing math longhand
"Friday's child is loving and giving."
pumpernickel-and-cheese appetizers
color wheels
a pole vaulter at the apex of the jump
breakers hammering a rocky coast
the contrast of dark brown and light blue
haiku poems: three lines unrhymed
Mister Milquetoast
Louboutin red soles

beating the weekend blues
take-a-number stores
fountain spray
an airtight rubber seal for a jar
loving-kindness
a setting of serenity and comfort
"Lola" (song)
wooden silverware instead of plastic at
     the coffee shop/deli
having a wry/rye sense of humor in a
     pumpernickel world
minute hands
scientific understanding
food gifts
reserve/junior varsity team practice
earbuds that do not pop out while
     exercising
conversation whipping gaily around a
     table like leaves in a wind
bentwood chairs and hanging lamps
what you would do with one extra hour
     a day
April evenings
the football huddle
herds of black-and-white cows drinking
     their reflections
supermarket aisles
pizza served on a large metal tray lined
     with white butcher's paper
a baby tooth under a pillow

Disneyland and Walt Disney World
finding out your IQ
taking the English Tunnel to the UK from
    France
figuring out how the hotel shower works
riding your bicycle to the store
cooking demonstrations
breath-catching evenings
"Well, I'm a dirty bird!"
Arctic poppies
buying your first expensive dress
raw barn siding
a car covered with bumper stickers
feeding ducks on the river
old rail fences wearily climbing the hill
flower-sprayed settings
saving an extra seat for yourself on the
    train or in a movie
European pro basketball
the best purchase you ever made
hotel and restaurant supply stores
watching Christmas specials
an ameliorative action
a place accessible only by bush plane
fog lathering up the stubbed field
warm food traveling through your throat
sunroofs
holiday fussing
dropping anchor
meditating in the bathtub

a sauce chef (saucier)

sloping expanses of white sand meeting the blue waters of an inland sea

coconut and Christmas palms, gardenias, ixora, crotons, and dieffenbachia

a crossover hit

artist studios open to the public

"better safe than sorry"

happy memories from childhood

guitar music at a coffeehouse

waves caught by a freeze and turned into a thick fringe of frosty lace on the rocky shore

when traveling, taking twice the money and half the clothes you think you'll need

the fuzzy texture of a peach

riotous coffee breaks

climbing into bed with your journal

in the pool where you least expect it, there will be a fish

cupping your eyes and other vision-improvement exercises

chilling out with friends

Care Bears

studying trees, buildings, scenery

a well-informed store clerk

remaining in a state of quiet repose

doing candles for every birthday

making clarinets squeak

petit dejeuner

remembering when there were no
 McDonald's

a unique synthesis of 3-D art, CG effects,
 architecture, artificial intelligence,
 sound effects, dramatic performances,
 music, storytelling, and interactivity

freestanding fireplaces

Ralph Waldo Emerson in matched
 volumes

Bob Hope, Bing Crosby, and Dorothy
 Lamour in the "Road" pictures

reminiscing

learning the ropes

stiff bristles sweeping

touching a cloud

nuthatches saying "yank"

being told you're beautiful when wearing
 a grungy T-shirt and jeans

commissioning a portrait

no two fingerprints being alike

too-hot-to-cook weather

a new mantra

the Coast Guard band

simple, satisfying tasks like sharpening
 pencils or clearing the clutter on
 your desk

a business incubator

knowing how to fold clothes for travel

ring-toss games

someone who ventures into unknown
territory and clears a path in the
wilderness for civilizations to follow,
who challenges accepted ideas about
what is possible and what can be
achieved

buffalo wings delivered to the dorm

buying something outrageous and then
something very practical to feel
vindicated

The Little Rascals (TV show)

cake made at the grocery store that has
the best icing

the vegetable gardener secretly wishing
for a frost

helping your child move into his first
apartment

laundry-sorting baskets

miles of toilet paper in trees

remembering all the sweet things
in your life

dulce de leche ice cream

sun infusing the atmosphere with
rich light

Kandinsky's *Farbstudie Quadrate*

predictive search

sneaking out of a place

knowing phone numbers by heart

a personalized gift

an English arboretum

a new coffee spot opening
ancient stone circles
being alone by the sea
wearing cleats
drafting tools
tweaking the school uniform to make it
     your own
ice-skating on ponds without skates
going back to an old favorite
white collars and cuffs and white sticking
     out under the sweater
brick porches
light meals
consideration for others
when the cat makes friends
Honolulu, in the southernmost U.S. state,
     Hawaii
magic carpets
floor-to-ceiling bookcases
experiencing synchronicity
foreign coins
homemade cards
the over-accessorizing of
     older women
a "winged" hairstyle after
     wearing a baseball cap
a happy, always crowded
     diner
getting accepted to the school you want
     to attend

pitching a tent on the beach
the tweet of a whistle
lighting up the place
the first day of sandals
a cold blue wash from the moon and
     stars polarizing the snowscape into
     a crosshatching of light and dark
getting away with things as much as
     possible
sketchbooks and charcoal
reading the fine print
defusing a bomb
high-definition television
bright rivers winding like silver threads
     through the soft, rich tapestries of
     growing fields
digging a moat
corrected astigmatism
the pendulum swinging and the cuckoo
     emerging from its ornate lodging
watching the Macy's parade balloons
     inflated at the American Museum of
     Natural History the night before
reverse phone directories
the smell of rain when the first drops
     come down and sink into the hot
     earth
the positive voice in your head
mistakes leading to epiphanies
the hum of window air conditioners

the dancing of fireflies as the moon rises

French fries, crisp and speckled with
shreds of skin

the days of the open range

finding the new *People* magazine at the
hairdresser

breeches, tall boots, and a riding jacket

arqo: the crossbar that turns an *R* into the
prescription symbol

a dessert called "Death by Chocolate"

making mushy Valentines for your lover

knowing how to play poker

writing punctuated with long pauses,
reflections, and ruminations

quiet feet

attempts to communicate with the
doughnut waitress on the other side
of the glass case

anniversary remembrances

Rice Krispies Marshmallow Treats

hilltop towns

finding loose change in your purse or
pocket—especially quarters

tiny percussive sounds

Louisiana: bayous, New Orleans, Creole
cooking, Mardi Gras

friends coming over

first lines of novels

secret gardens glimpsed through tall
windows

attending a production of *Messiah*
lemon sherbet
deep-sixing a bad idea
your face to the window, inhaling the
    scenery
the 23 fruit flavors in Dr Pepper
St. Louis, Missouri: Gateway to the West
a comic in a club, warming up an audience
cooking without a recipe
being in tune with nature
patio parties
knowing right where to look for
    something
toddlers' vocabulary
how you would spend a month of vacation
sponsoring a Little League team
the gift of every day
seeking others' advice
almanac forecasts
the sunny side of living
an island accessible only by boat
nature undefiled
the soft interior of a loaf of bread
wrought-iron fences
a buttermilk sky
window glass
discovering an explanation for something,
    like Asian flush syndrome
hands on a ship
making your own pizza

a stamp for printing your name on brown
bags, etc.
ordering the mind, replenishing the heart,
finding yourself again
small at-home dinners
a stormy weekend to get reacquainted
with the most comfortable chair in
the house
the Smart Car (1998)
needing a hug, a cuddle, and love
Earth, a milky-blue marble against the
jeweler's velvet space
swimming laps at the YMCA
the sweet bass accompaniment of
burbling spaghetti
snow-lathered cars being shaved
public transportation
water rights
overtipping
a suit made to order
ice-cream dispensers
something falling neatly
into place
someone levitated by a magician
making up songs, both lyric and theme
a romantic message posted on a
scoreboard
wearing real jewelry
moving on from your to-do to your want-
to-do list

five-card stud

agreeing with anybody bigger than
    you are

finding the video/DVD you wanted,
    even though you couldn't remember
    the title

the resident cat on the porch rail

computer scientists

butter cookies and milk

a view of the river

angel hair pasta

salt-and-pepper shakers collected over
    the years

rewards for using your credit card

saving up for a house

teriyaki steaks

chef salad

getting off an airplane after a long flight

ducks parading on a pond

the atom, the smallest unit of matter
    that retains the characteristics of
    an element, and the molecule, the
    smallest unit of matter that retains
    the characteristics of a compound

thumbing the spout of a drinking fountain

souvenirs on the road: snow globes,
    beaded belts, mini license plates,
    pens with figures that move, bumper
    stickers, refrigerator magnets, pins,
    hats, patches, mugs, pennants

May's great green canopy spreading along
    every tree-lined street
singing all the hymns in church
room-service food brought on a cart
watching a children's program
sitting cross-legged in the window
McGuffey's six reader-primers
twilight lingering at the end of the day like
    a promise
a cat purring
being an anonymous donor
the smell of aerosol hair spray
writing at dawn or when everybody else
    goes to sleep
Heath ice-cream bars
the best climbing rocks
savoir faire
touring local industries
drawer dividers
melon season
Coke vs. Pepsi
doll strollers
aerial mapping
the weight of coconut bowls
hearing the high school marching band
    practice
"You are what you read."
driving alone
"welcome home" flowers
foamy clouds

someone to read your mind
well-written instruction booklets
beef brisket, barbecued or smothered in
    liquid smoke
the detector in an aspirin that tells it
    exactly what part of the body to go to
"The First Noel" (carol)
raising kids
successful damage control
a candle burning under a vegetable grater
the least attractive side of a Christmas
    tree that ends up facing the wall
taking a hike
an outfitted picnic hamper
finding a perfectly ripe mango
making and coloring maps
petting zoos
paying close attention to everything
TV bloopers and movie outtakes
ancient ruins
to be engrossed by something outside
    yourself
individual cartoon frames
half the world living in five countries
hanging in there
savoring the elemental
teenagers who smile at and acknowledge
    older people
borrowing a hand truck
donating blood

examining your conscience
a landscape sprinkled with lakes rimmed
    by thick forest and soaring bluffs
a Thomas Edison Ediphone
Apple and Microsoft
fireside tray suppers
your fortune read from coffee grounds
adding a touch of charades to your
    conversation
gray New England winter mornings
broiling to perfection
the cheering of the crowd
successfully moving all your clothes
    from the washer to the dryer
    without dropping anything
word of mouse
ivory figurines
a broiler that cooks both sides of a steak
    at once in an oven
the supermarket meat department
a tired Santa
the theme song to *Masterpiece Mystery*
    on PBS
baking your own pound cake
approval
exercising at the Y
the difference between nuts and seeds
journals transformed by repeated and
    fond use
learning to lay a fire

the smell of old school buildings
a really clean shave
camellias like starched organdy
steak medallions au poivre
rock gardens
joking to lighten the mood
bell towers
crazy New York taxis
a favorite food you cook in home
    economics or a useful project you
    complete in shop/woodworking class
active leisure
meditation retreats at Spirit Rock or Kripalu
hearts warming when friends meet
the back roads in the Hamptons
the last shy bloomings of wild rose in
    already fading brambles
talking to the animals at the zoo
tiring yourself out
thwarting troublemakers
leaving the water running while brushing
    your teeth, sometimes
congeniality
people who bob up and down in the ocean
    trying to stay dry above the waist
stacking books by the bed in the order
    you want to read them
a season for loving and remembering
always wanting to be a kid when you
    grew up

Italian marbled paper
medicine kits
a showoff
the feel of a scarf against the neck
an organ loft
Mom food: meat loaf, macaroni and
    cheese, fish sticks, spaghetti, chicken
    pot pie, ham and scalloped potatoes
reading Dickens
getting what you want and what you need
    at the same time
newspaper publishing
the Final Four of the NCAA basketball
    tournament
waiting for the light to turn green when
    you've spotted an empty parking
    space across the intersection
a big night out
a rag rug, a boot box, a cat to sleep in the
    wash basket
the reaction of a teenager when the
    phone rings
Waldorf salad
learning to love and appreciate easy-
    listening music
babies' silverware
sybarite: anyone who loves luxury and
    self-indulgence
old records
anything yellow

plump channel quilting
the head-for-the-beach-anyway plan
one minute equaling 15 double-spaced
    typewritten lines in a speech
conjugal bliss
a toasted, buttered hot dog bun
nest-building
"Your guess is as good as mine."
a table between two comfy reading chairs
pints of pork fried rice with duck sauce
calamine lotion
taking a class in something totally
    esoteric
daily reminders
an epic diary entry, detailing love life,
    career, friendship
"God Rest Ye Merry Gentlemen" (carol)
In and Out trays
drawbridges and moats
saying something nice
fringe benefits
writing dedications for books and articles
a weekend away for your anniversary
when your cat had kittens
a blanket of vapor on a still summer day
Dr. Scholl's exercise sandals
poetry reading
"Work is love made visible." (Kahlil
    Gibran)
mastering the perfect vinaigrette

Thoreau—the patron saint of the written
    journal
seeing the unexpected and reveling in the
    incongruities
being as giddy as a cat on catnip
the opportunity to see how a person
    operates
fighting global warming with good gas
    mileage
the slow tumble of a dust bunny under the
    dining table
taking local honey to quell a spring allergy
discovering "how things work"
Weather Channel's Local on the 8s
hearing a song you liked so
        much in high school, but
        haven't heard in years
log cabins
how good it feels to change into
        comfortable nightclothes
a cloud forest—a tropical forest atop
        coastal mountains
visiting the Rome Catacombs carved
        in soft tufa rock
the sun filling your bones with light
a bike ride on a country lane
scribbling comments in the margins
        of books
sizing up the real-estate market
noticing the color of the snow

the Scoville Scale for chile peppers

something you say that wasn't intended to
be funny, but is anyway

the magic of improving your posture

a desert dotted with cactus and red-clay
paths

forays into Barbie Dream House decor

a conversation with a historical society
curator

when the cat sneaks onto the bed to sleep
while you're out

reupholstering the interior of an old VW

the nurturing side of your personality

finding out the cause of something

that outfit you always feel confident and
comfortable in

needle-threading and thimbles

the discovery of light in a dark situation

letting the guy in a hurry cut in front of
you in line

reflecting on all that is good in your life

never taking a course from a professor
who wrote the textbook

south-facing windows providing heat
in the winter

someone who can rebuild a
transmission

the 21 badges needed to become
an Eagle Scout

a need for and a confidence in solitude

the impossibility of folding a piece of
    paper in half more than seven times
using this book for discovering and
    generating ideas for artworks
the koalas in Barnum's Animal Crackers
elevators being the safest form of
    transportation
burning 100 calories an hour just sitting
keeping your own list of things to be
    happy about
rare-book rooms in the great libraries
beef bologna
clutch purses
bon voyage gifts
mock turtlenecks
tavern firelight and playing parlor games
big beach balls
Seriously?
pet portraits
an intimate dinner
    for two on the
    coffee table
a hole-in-one in
    miniature golf
wondering why *abbreviation* is such
    a long word
baked-potato jackets
dozens of places to curl up with a book

ABOUT THE AUTHOR

Barbara Ann Kipfer is a lexicographer and author. Her works include *The Wish List*, *8,789 Words of Wisdom*, *Self-Meditation*, *Instant Karma*, and *The Order of Things*, as well as thesauri, reference books, spiritually themed books, and other list books. She holds doctorates in linguistics, archaeology, and Buddhist studies and has worked for companies such as Temnos, Google, Ask, Ask Jeeves, Dictionary.com, General Electric Research, IBM Research, Idealab, Knowledge Adventure, and Wolfram|Alpha. Her website is thingstobehappyabout.com.